T0348521

Inclusivity in Dentistry: Environments of Belonging and Equity

Editors

LESLIE R. HALPERN
LINDA M. KASTE
JANET H. SOUTHERLAND

DENTAL CLINICS OF NORTH AMERICA

www.dental.theclinics.com

January 2025 • Volume 69 • Number 1

ELSEVIER

1600 John F. Kennedy Boulevard • Suite 1800 • Philadelphia, Pennsylvania, 19103-2899

http://www.dental.theclinics.com

DENTAL CLINICS OF NORTH AMERICA Volume 69, Number 1
January 2025 ISSN 0011-8532, ISBN: 978-0-443-31410-0

Editor: John Vassallo; j.vassallo@elsevier.com
Developmental Editor: Akshay Samson

Dental Clinics of North America (ISSN 0011-8532) is published quarterly by Elsevier Inc., 360 Park Avenue South, New York, NY 10010-1710. Months of issue are January, April, July, and October. Business and Editorial Offices: 1600 John F. Kennedy Boulevard, Suite 1800, Philadelphia, PA 19103-2899. Periodicals postage paid at New York, NY and additional mailing offices. Subscription prices are $343.00 per year (domestic individuals), $100.00 per year (domestic students/residents), $408.00 per year (Canadian individuals), $100.00 per year (Canadian students/residents) $477.00 per year (international individuals), and $200.00 per year (international students/residents). For institutional access pricing please contact Customer Service via the contact information below. International air speed delivery is included in all *Clinics* subscription prices. All prices are subject to change without notice. Orders, claims, and journal inquiries: Please visit our Support Hub page https://service.elsevier.com for assistance.

Reprints. For copies of 100 or more, of articles in this publication, please contact the Commercial Reprints Department, Elsevier Inc., 360 Park Avenue South, New York, NY 10010-1710. Tel.: 212-633-3874; Fax: 212-633-3820; E-mail: reprints@elsevier.com.

The Dental Clinics of North America is covered in *MEDLINE/PubMed (Index Medicus), Current Contents/Clinical Medicine, ISI/BIOMED* and *Cinahl.*

Contributors

EDITORS

LESLIE R. HALPERN, DDS, MD, PhD, MPH, FACS, FICD
Professor, Section Chief/Program Director, Oral and Maxillofacial Surgery Residency, Department of Dental Medicine, New York Medical College, NYC Health + Hospitals/ Metropolitan, Valhalla, New York

LINDA M. KASTE, DDS, MS, PhD, FAADOCR, FICD
Professor, Department of Oral Biology, University of Illinois Chicago College of Dentistry, Chicago, Illinois

JANET H. SOUTHERLAND, DDS, MPH, PhD
Vice Chancellor of Academic Affairs and Chief Academic Officer; Professor, Oral and Maxillofacial Surgery; Institutional Research Officer; Interim Dean of School of Dentistry, LSU Health Sciences Center New Orleans, New Orleans, Louisiana

AUTHORS

KENDRA M. BARRIER, PhD, MSN, RN, CNE
Associate Dean for Diversity, Equity, and Inclusion, Assistant Professor of Clinical Nursing, School of Nursing, LSU Health Sciences Center New Orleans, New Orleans, Louisiana

KATE L. BLALACK, MHR, MLIS, CA, DAS
Associate Librarian, Digital Repositories, Library Applications Management, Hesburgh Libraries, University of Notre Dame, Notre Dame, Indiana

TAMMI O. BYRD, RDH
CEO/Clinical Director, Health Promotion Specialists, Portable Community Clinic, South Carolina, Columbia, South Carolina

KENDALL M. CAMPBELL, MD, FAAFP
Chair and Professor, Department of Family Medicine, University of Texas Medical Branch, Galveston, Texas

BENITA N. CHATMON, PhD, MSN, RN, CNE
Associate Professor, Assistant Dean for Clinical Nursing Education, School of Nursing, LSU Health Sciences Center New Orleans, New Orleans, Louisiana

ELISA M. CHÁVEZ, DDS
Professor, Diagnostic Sciences; Director, Pacific Center for Equity in Oral Health Care, University of the Pacific, Arthur A. Dugoni School of Dentistry, San Francisco, California

ALISON F. DOUBLEDAY, MA, MS, PhD
Director of Faculty Development, Associate Professor, Department of Oral Medicine and Diagnostic Sciences, College of Dentistry, University of Illinois Chicago, Chicago, Illinois

ELEANOR FLEMING, PhD, DDS, MPH, FICD
Clinical Associate Professor, University of Maryland School of Dentistry, Baltimore, Maryland

SARA C. GORDON, DDS, MS
Associate Dean for Academic Affairs, Professor, Department of Oral Medicine, School of Dentistry, University of Washington, Seattle, Washington

COLIN M. HALEY, DDS, MED, MHA
Clinical Associate Professor, Department of Oral Medicine and Diagnostic Sciences, College of Dentistry, University of Illinois Chicago, Chicago, Illinois

LESLIE R. HALPERN, DDS, MD, PhD, MPH, FACS, FICD
Professor, Section Chief/Program Director, Oral and Maxillofacial Surgery Residency, Department of Dental Medicine, New York Medical College, NYC Health + Hospitals/Metropolitan, Valhalla, New York

SHULAMITE S. HUANG, PhD
Assistant Professor, Department of Epidemiology and Health Promotion, New York University College of Dentistry, New York, New York

LINDA M. KASTE, DDS, MS, PhD, FAADOCR, FICD
Professor, Department of Oral Biology, University of Illinois Chicago College of Dentistry, Chicago, Illinois

MELANIE MORRIS, LCSW
Assistant Professor, Department of Comprehensive Care, Tufts University School of Dental Medicine, Boston, Massachusetts

CHARLES P. MOUTON, MD, MS, MBA
Executive Vice President, Provost, and Executive Dean, Professor, Family Medicine, School of Medicine, University of Texas Medical Branch, Galveston, Texas

HERMINIO L. PEREZ, DMD, MBA, EdD
Assistant Dean of Student Affairs, Diversity and Inclusion, Rutgers School of Dental Medicine, Newark, New Jersey

DEMETRIUS J. PORCHE, DNS, PhD, APRN, FACHE, FAANP, FAAN
Dean and Professor, LSU Health Sciences Center New Orleans, School of Nursing, New Orleans, Louisiana

JOANNE L. PRASAD, DDS, MPH
Assistant Dean for Academic Affairs, Associate Professor, Departments of Oral and Craniofacial Sciences, and Diagnostic Sciences, University of Pittsburgh School of Dental Medicine, Pittsburgh, Pennsylvania

MARY K. ROJEK, PhD
Director of Faculty Affairs and Development, University of South Carolina School of Medicine Greenville, Greenville, South Carolina

STEFANIE L. RUSSELL, DDS, MPH, PhD
Associate Professor, Department of Pediatric Dentistry and Community Dentistry, Rutgers School of Dental Medicine, Newark, New Jersey

JANET H. SOUTHERLAND, DDS, MPH, PhD
Vice Chancellor of Academic Affairs and Chief Academic Officer; Professor, Oral and Maxillofacial Surgery; Institutional Research Officer; Interim Dean of School of Dentistry, LSU Health Sciences Center New Orleans, New Orleans, Louisiana

SILVIA SPIVAKOVSKI, DDS
Clinical Professor, Department of Oral and Maxillofacial Pathology, Radiology and Medicine, New York University College of Dentistry, New York, New York

STEPH TUAZON, LCSW
Practicum Education Consultant, Luskin School of Public Affairs - Social Welfare, School of Dentistry, Special Patient Care, University of California, Los Angeles, Los Angeles, California

CHRISTINE WIESELER, PhD
Assistant Professor, Department of Philosophy, Santa Clara University, Santa Clara, California

JANET A. YELLOWITZ, DMD, MPH
Associate Professor, Director, Geriatric Dentistry, University of Maryland School of Dentistry, Baltimore, Maryland

JUDY CHIA-CHUN YUAN, DDS, MS, MAS, FACP
Professor, Department of Restorative Dentistry, University of Illinois Chicago College of Dentistry, Chicago, Illinois

CANDACE ZIGLOR, DSW, LMSW
Clinical Assistant Professor, University of Detroit Mercy, School of Dentistry, Detroit, Michigan

Contents

Inclusion is an essential part of diversity, equity, and inclusion. Dentistry's history has been such that the profession has experienced inclusion and exclusion, sometimes by choice and sometimes by the actions of others. This study reviews the concept of inclusion in the context of the current need to create inclusive environments for a workforce that is culturally and structurally sound to serve all patients, including the underrepresented or marginalized, in integrated health care. Additionally, this article serves as an introductory roadmap to the papers in this Dental Clinics of North America issue discussing components of inclusivity in dentistry.

Inclusive language in dentistry is essential for delivering high-quality, equitable care that respects and empathizes with patients from diverse backgrounds. It involves using language that avoids exclusion and bias, focusing on person-first terms, and understanding the preferences of individuals and communities. This approach not only promotes health equity and belonging but also strengthens trust and communication between providers and patients and among members of the dental health care team. Education, training, and consistent deliberate practice in inclusive language among health care professionals are crucial for integrating these principles into oral health care.

Dentistry has traditionally been male-dominated in North America, although "primary care" dentistry disciplines, including dental public health (DPH), have greater gender equity than other areas. However, gender gaps are likely to persist, specifically in academia. As an example of the measurement of inclusion, we sought to identify gender equity in authorship in publications in DPH and epidemiology over six years. We found that while women occupied first and second authorship positions, men dominated the senior author position. Evaluating gender in authorship provides valuable information on inclusion and the movement toward achieving gender equity in dental public health.

This article represents a prologue of the discussion of the article "Models of DEIB: Part II–Exploring Models of Inclusion from other Health Professions for Dentistry". It explores existing practices and philosophies from other disciplines that could be applied toward creating environments of inclusion and belonging in dentistry. The primary focus here is to provide an opportunity for the dental profession to leverage knowledge and experiences from other health professions to enhance and expand inclusion efforts and provide enhance engagement at all levels.

This study describes examples of models and frameworks from other professions that could be applied toward creating environments of inclusion and belonging in dentistry. Examples are provided of activities, frameworks, and models that can serve to launch similar activities within dentistry. Selected models of inclusion from library science, medicine, nursing, dental hygiene, and social work can be used by the dental profession to help make definitive strides in the inclusion arena to combat challenges of access and inequitable oral health status.

Dentistry has faced, and continues to face, challenges in expanding its ranks to include diverse, especially minoritized, people. American Indian/Alaska Native, Hispanic, and Black representation, for example, has not grown significantly in dentistry. Although dental schools have an accreditation standard to be humanistic environments, it is not clear that dental schools have climates that are functionally inclusive of minoritized people—whether for patients, the student body, staff members, faculty members or leadership. For the profession to advance oral health equity, intentional efforts are needed in education and across the full dental workforce.

The United States (US) population and the dental workforce are becoming increasingly diverse. Characteristics of the April 2024 cohort of the 65 permanently named deans at Commission on Dental Accreditation-recognized US dental schools show the most diversity among deans yet. This cohort demonstrates increases in the representation of women and non-Whites, as well as substantial number of those who are internationally dental school-trained. This article explores individual and dental school characteristics for these deans through an inclusive lens. The "30% Solution" is considered as a critical mass benchmark for achieving meaningful representation of diversity and inclusivity among these deans.

Biomedical and structural factors impact oral health for people with intellectual and developmental disabilities (IDD). The onset of age prevalent chronic diseases and conditions can result in new cognitive or physical disabilities leaving individuals with IDD to contend with ageism as well as ableism and further exclusion from the oral health care systems. Environments and attitudes that inform how health care systems are built and maintained significantly impact quality of life and outcomes, more than the fact of being disabled or old. Understanding and easing the transitions that lay ahead of individuals aging with IDD will come from an interprofessional inclusive approach.

Sex and gender are essential components of person-centered care. This article presents and discusses four important tenets regarding sex and gender health that should be incorporated into dental education and oral health care to foster inclusivity and improve care for all patients, including a sex and gender-diverse patient population.

The article explores the evolution and significance of mentoring, drawing from Greek mythology, particularly the story of Odysseus and Mentor. It defines mentoring as a developmental relationship beneficial for mentees, mentors, and organizations, particularly in academia and health care. The article covers various mentoring models, including traditional, peer, reverse, group, e-mentoring, and the mosaic model, emphasizing inclusivity and cultural responsiveness. The social construct framework and the inclusive mentorship approach are highlighted, addressing barriers faced by underrepresented groups. The importance of understanding social and cultural identities for effective mentoring, especially in dental education, is highlighted.

Inclusivity in Dentistry: Environments of Belonging and Equity

DENTAL CLINICS OF NORTH AMERICA

SERIES OF RELATED INTEREST

Atlas of the Oral and Maxillofacial Surgery Clinics
https://www.oralmaxsurgeryatlas.theclinics.com/

Oral and Maxillofacial Surgery Clinics
https://www.oralmaxsurgery.theclinics.com/

THE CLINICS ARE AVAILABLE ONLINE!
Access your subscription at:
www.theclinics.com

Preface

Inclusivity in Dentistry: Environments of Belonging and Equity

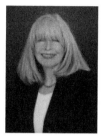

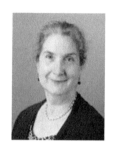

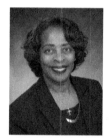

Leslie R. Halpern, DDS, MD, PhD, MPH, FACS, FICD

Linda M. Kaste, DDS, MS, PhD, FAADOCR, FICD

Janet H. Southerland, DDS, MPH, PhD

Editors

The ethnic, racial, ability, aging, cultural, and linguistic diversity of the US population is increasing significantly, as seen especially over the past several decades and reaching into the future. Correspondingly, diversity, equity, inclusion, and belonging (DEIB) and justice and accessibility are topics that merit recognition in all components of health care. Dental educators and clinicians need to be both aware and skilled to enable the promotion of inclusive, engaging, and productive environments for patients as well as for the dental workforce.

The argument for inclusion to broaden DEIB in the dental profession is vital, as inclusion provides the foundation for building leadership, cultural humility within a humanistic environment, engagement, social justice, and more, such as to incentivize successful careers. Inclusivity provides the "glue" to align diversity, equity, accessibility, and justice as well as the sense of belonging starting from within academic institutions as vehicles that reach into health care and community. Oral health care providers must reflect and respect the diverse populations for whom they are serving. Although intuitive, no model or set of criteria in dentistry fully exemplifies this concept. Posing roadmaps to enhance strategies for the education and practice of dentistry enables guides for transformational change in dental education, patient care, and population health. The intent of this issue of *Dental Clinics of North America* is to provide sketches of such roadmaps. This issue delves into topics that are elements of inclusion as support for dentistry in traveling these roads.

Each of the articles in this issue contributes at least one aspect to the groundwork of inclusivity in dentistry. The first half provides overarching perspectives on inclusivity, starting with an overview introduction in the article "The "I" in Diversity, Equity, and

Dent Clin N Am 69 (2025) xi–xiii
https://doi.org/10.1016/j.cden.2024.09.001
0011-8532/25/© 2024 Published by Elsevier Inc.

dental.theclinics.com

Inclusion: The Challenge of Inclusivity in Dentistry". The article "Inclusive Language to Support Health Equity and Belonging in Dentistry" introduces the reader to the principles of language that serve to create an empathetic environment that acknowledges and supports health equity and a sense of belonging. The article "A Measure of Inclusion: Women as Authors in Oral Epidemiology and Dental Public Health, 2017–2022" discusses measuring inclusion with the example of gender equity in authorship. The articles "Models of Diversity, Equity, Inclusion, and Belonging: Part I—Approaches to Inclusion from Other Health Professions for Consideration by Dentistry" and "Models of Diversity, Equity, Inclusion, and Belonging: Part II—Exploring Models of Inclusion from Other Health Professions for Dentistry" in two parts provide overviews of models for inclusion in DEIB from other health professions of medicine, nursing, dental hygiene, library sciences, and social work. The authors describe expanding efforts to embrace inclusivity across the dental profession by hypothesizing collaborative efforts not just within the profession but also in conjunction with colleagues across the health professions.

The second half of the articles provides additional insight into applications for dentistry. The article "Advancing Dentistry Through Respectful Inclusion: A Focus on Racial Inequities" confers the advancing of dentistry through respectful inclusion by describing intentional efforts needed in education and across the full dental workforce. In the article "United States Dental School Deans' Characteristics Through an Inclusive Lens," the dean-level leadership at US dental schools is reviewed at the current status against the "30% Solution" considered a critical mass benchmark to achieve meaningful, sustainable representation of diversity and inclusivity. The examination of ageism, ableism, and inclusivity occurs for individuals aging with intellectual and developmental disabilities in the article "Ageism and Ableism in Individuals Aging with Intellectual and Developmental Disabilities." The article "Sex and Gender Health Education Tenets: An Essential Paradigm for Inclusivity in Dentistry" incorporates consideration of sex and gender health tenets into dental education for oral health care that fosters inclusivity and optimal care for all patients. The article "Inclusivity in Mentorship: Shifting Paradigms of Inclusion in Dental Education" provides closure in this series with the review of dental education with consideration of a "mosaic" mentoring model through which academic dentistry can be a more inclusive environment.

We are privileged to provide the issue "Inclusivity in Dentistry: Environments of Belonging and Equity" with its focus on evolving concepts of inclusivity. As educators and practitioners in their respective disciplines and professions, in and outside of dentistry, the authors provide key commentary by bringing forward a thought-provoking series of roadmaps to enhance strategies for inclusivity in the dental profession. We greatly appreciate their essential contributions to this issue and to the progress on inclusivity in dentistry. In addition, we wish to extend our thanks to Mr John Vassallo, Editor of *Dental Clinics of North America*, for his support and encouragement of this project. Our relationships with colleagues across many professions embody the definition of inclusion and belonging across the spectrum of oral health care. We are inspired by the possibilities to continue highlighting the importance of inclusion in oral health.

Leslie R. Halpern, DDS, MD, PhD, MPH, FACS, FICD
Oral and Maxillofacial Surgery Residency
New York Medical College
100 Woods Road
Valhalla, NY 10595, USA

Linda M. Kaste, DDS, MS, PhD, FAADOCR, FICD
Department of Oral Biology
University of Illinois Chicago
College of Dentistry
801 South Paulina Street
Chicago, IL 60612, USA

Janet H. Southerland, DDS, MPH, PhD
LSU Health Sciences Center, New Orleans
433 Bolivar Street
New Orleans, LA 70112, USA

E-mail addresses:
halpernl@nychhc.org (L.R. Halpern)
kaste@uic.edu (L.M. Kaste)
jsouther@lhshsc.edu (J.H. Southerland)

The "I" in Diversity, Equity, and Inclusion
The Challenge of Inclusivity in Dentistry

Leslie R. Halpern, DDS, MD, PhD, MPH, FICD[a],*,
Linda M. Kaste, DDS, MS, PhD, FAADOCR, FICD[b],
Janet H. Southerland, DDS, MPH, PhD[c]

KEYWORDS

- Diversity • Equity • Inclusion • Intersectionality • Inclusive practice
- Inclusive strategies • Interprofessional relations • Dentistry

KEY POINTS

- Inclusion is an essential part of diversity, equity, and inclusion as well as with the broader concepts captured with accessibility, belonging, and justice.
- Imagery for the population perspective in the United States for inclusion has moved from the melting pot where everyone was to adapt to be the same to the mixed salad or chili where separate contributions are recognizable but work together to make the best whole.
- The impact of inclusion ranges from the individual to the professional and population communities.
- Elements for dentistry need to be developed, to have the realization for optimal health care for all, so that other aspects of health care recognize the requirement of bidirectional inclusion of dentistry and oral health. Dentistry must be at the table and serve as a leader in inclusion among the health care professions.

INTRODUCTION

Inclusion as the last word listed in the context of diversity, equity, and inclusion (DEI) may be the word with the least attention paid to it. As solutions are sought for inequities and disparities, particularly related to health status and health care access in the United States, the importance of inclusion rises. Additionally, the importance of inclusion is magnified by seeing that it applies to everyone. A variety of definitions have arisen for inclusion or inclusivity (see **Box 1** for examples).[1–7] This study serves as an

[a] Department of Dental Medicine/WMC/New York Medical College, Macey Pavilion, 100 Woods Road, Valhalla, NY 10583, USA; [b] Department of Oral Biology, University of Illinois Chicago College of Dentistry, 801 South Paulina Street, Chicago, IL 60612, USA; [c] LSU Health Sciences Center, New Orleans, 433 Bolivar Street, New Orleans, LA 70112, USA
* Corresponding author.
E-mail address: halpernl@nychhc.org

Dent Clin N Am 69 (2025) 1–15
https://doi.org/10.1016/j.cden.2024.08.006
0011-8532/25/© 2024 Elsevier Inc. All rights reserved, including those for text and data mining, AI training, and similar technologies.
dental.theclinics.com

Box 1
Examples of definitions for inclusion in the context of diversity, equity, and inclusion

American Dental Association[1]
   Inclusion: Enables us to strive to have all people represented and included and make everyone feel a sense of belonging, not only for their abilities, but also for their unique qualities and perspectives.

American Dental Education Association[2]
   Inclusion: The practice of leveraging diversity to ensure individuals can fully participate and perform at their best. Inclusion is shared responsibility of everyone within the community. An inclusive environment values differences rather than suppressing them; promotes respect, success, and a sense of belonging; and fosters well-being through policies, programs, practices, learning, and dialogue.

FDI World Dental Federation[3,4]
   National Health Policy[3]: The new definition of oral health adopted by the FDI World Dental Federation General Assembly in 2016 has laid the framework to allow the profession to reflect on what oral health encompasses and its implication for national oral health policies. Further, this definition, which was approved by consensus by FDI constituents, favors the inclusion of oral health in all health-related policies ....

Our Values[4]
   Culture of inclusiveness: We deliberately and meaningfully engage and seek representation from the diverse range of oral health professionals and the communities and individuals they serve. This is paramount to achieving our mission.

International Association for Dental Research[5]
   SCIENCE POLICY: Diversity, Equity, Inclusion, Accessibility, and Belonging Statement:
   Inclusion is the recognition, appreciation, and use of the talents and skills of all backgrounds by creating a welcoming environment through the proactive identification and removal of the barriers that impede the success of all.

National Academies of Sciences, Engineering, and Medicine[6]
   Ending Unequal Treatment: Strategies to Achieve Equitable Health care and Optimal Health for All.
   Inclusion: Efforts used to embrace differences; also used to describe how much each person feels welcomed, respected, supported, and valued in a given context.

[White House] Executive Order (14035) on Diversity, Equity, Inclusion, and Accessibility in the Federal Workforce[7]

The term "inclusion" means the recognition, appreciation, and use of the talents and skills of employees of all backgrounds.

---

introduction to issues around inclusion for the dental profession and the discussions developed further in the accompanying articles in this issue of Dental Clinics of North America on Inclusivity in Dentistry: Environments of Belonging and Equity.

The diversity of the US population is increasing significantly. The projected trends are such that by 2034, adults over 65 years old will outnumber children under the age of 18 years, and as of 2045, non-Hispanic Whites will no longer be in the majority.[8] Traditionally, the trajectory of health care providers was hoped to "mirror" the population demographics. However, the reflection has not been optimal. Risk predictors for health disparities have tipped the scale in terms of health care inequity as evidenced by increases in the lack of access to care, especially for historically underserved and marginalized groups who are susceptible to significant health conditions and risk of mortality.[9,10]

The considerations and recognitions of the importance of DEI are complex and are not new as confirmed by decades of inequity and injustice. Some reflect on the civil rights movement in the 1960s as being the initiator of DEI.[11] Yet orientation to this time as the starting point reinforces thoughts about just what are the definitions and contexts of DEI use, as it seems that the very premise of the founding of the United States was on equity.[12]

Nevertheless, evolution is happening in the United States; dentistry is in it and needs to embrace the changes and engage to optimize the effectiveness of the profession. One question to ask is what fits best for the US population or the dental workforce as an analogy: a melting pot,[13] a mixed salad,[14] chili,[15] or a boiling pot[16–18]?

The diversification of the US population is directly relevant to dentistry for addressing whether the dental workforce reflects the patient population. Contrasts of the components of dentistry viewed from first-year dental students to the dental workforce against the US population yield interesting and encouraging observations on the progress being made at the dental student entry level against the significant gaps from the perspectives of the workforce and dental school deans that are disproportionately non-Hispanic White male individuals (**Fig. 1**).[19–23]

A dynamic reflection on the desire to have a convenient term for seeking priorities and actions is that of the number of acronyms that have emerged. DEI has been expanded to consider other values, such as diversity, equity, inclusion and belonging (DEIB) with the addition of belonging, and justice, equity, diversity, inclusion (JEDI) or equity, diversity, justice, inclusion (EDIJ) when considering justice. The Federal Workforce adds another concept that of accessibility in its use of diversity, equity, inclusion, and accessibility in the June 25, 2021, Executive Order 14035.[24] Interesting, in addition to government and academia, a consistent driver of trying to figure out what works best regarding the impact of inclusion and diversity is business and business is an important element of the dental profession.[25–27]

The US Surgeon General (1982–1989) C. Everett Koop observed a strong tie between dentistry and medicine. "You are not healthy without good oral health" is widely cited in dentistry,[28–30] while similar value does not always seem to be placed on its importance by medicine as the quote could not be found among Web sites with top quotes from and tributes to Surgeon General Koop.[31,32]

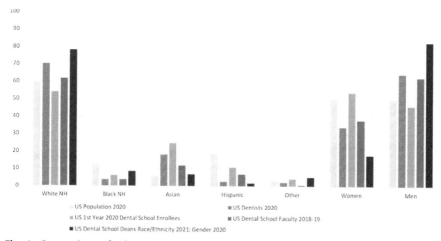

Fig. 1. Comparison of selected demographic percentages circa 2020 by total population,[19] dentist workforce,[19] first year dental students,[20] dental school faculty members,[21] and dental school deans.[22,23]

INDEPENDENCE VERSUS INCLUSION: A BRIEF REVIEW OF DENTAL HISTORY AND DENTAL PROFESSIONALS

Dentistry as a profession has been reacting to inclusion in the context of whether the mouth belongs to the body for centuries. Splits are notable from the roles of the barber surgeons and establishment of the first dental college as measures of what medicine did not incorporate that became the features of the evolving profession dentistry, potentially using a collaborative practice model.[33] The concept of collaborative, inclusive health care has taken a long time to manifest and has not yet been fully realized. See **Box 2** for selected supplemental readings on broad societal perspectives on inclusion and belonging. The paradigm shift that has taken place in health care toward a more holistic and inclusive care model involving all systems of the body and the mouth is also required to address disparities that continue to produce inequities seen in oral health outcomes.

The profession of dentistry has some similarities to other health care professions but also has distinct differences. In the United States and Europe, dentistry has experienced exclusion from broader health system discussions and decisions. Such seems possibly attributable to the profession evolving from a trade and the solo expectation that dentistry takes care of teeth. The historic medical view of teeth has been that teeth are disposable, and it is inevitable to have them all lost, more of a nuisance than an essential contribution to overall function.[33] The evolution of other components of health care circa other body parts, eyes and ears, or heart, for example, has gone differently. Perhaps dentistry's history would be different if the original view of the body part in question was the mouth rather than the tooth. What if an early medical thought that has been attributed to Hippocrates of "all disease begins in the gut" had been more inclusive of the mouth being the portal to the gut? A recent review of the human microbiome is motivating for inclusive perspectives for health across the body.[34] This suggested approach to an inclusive perspective has taken a long time to arrive and the story continues to be written. Dentistry has often been challenged by dynamics within the dental team, the medical system, and oral health disparities to name a few aspects. Working more diligently on achieving inclusivity at all levels will be instrumental in addressing the most glaring of the challenges that of improved oral health outcomes across the lifespan.

Box 2
Selected supplemental readings on perspectives on inclusion

2000 Paulo Freire. Pedagogy of the Oppressed: 50th Anniversary Edition. Bloomsbury Academic: New York.

2017 No Health without Oral Health: How the dental community can leverage the NCD agenda to deliver on the 2030 Sustainable Development Goals. FDI World Dental Federation: Geneva-Cointrin, Switzerland.

2019 Tomas Chamorro-Premuzic. Why Do So Many Incompetent Men Become Leaders? (and how to fix it). Harvard Business Review Press: Boston, Massachusetts.

2020 Stefanie K. Johnson. Inclusify: The Power of Uniqueness and Belonging to Build Innovative Teams. Harper Business/Harper Collins Publishers: New York.

2020 Isabel Wilkerson. Caste: The Origins of Our Discontents. Random House: New York.

2024 National Academies of Sciences, Engineering, and Medicine. Ending Unequal Treatment: Strategies to Achieve Equitable Health Care and Optimal Health for All. The National Academies Press: Washington, DC.

DENTAL PROFESSIONALS CHALLENGED WITH INCLUSION

Within dentistry, several notable challenges of inclusion persist within the profession across professional components. Several examples are provided here. The first explores the question of "Does oral surgery 'belong' to medicine or dentistry?" Oral surgeons walk on the border of these 2 professions, with many having both medical and dental doctoral degrees, albeit the pathway for oral maxillofacial surgery's inclusion in surgery has been a bit of a circular path (**Box 3**) for historic perspective from the training program at Harvard University, the first university-affiliated dental school.[35,36] The trade-offs might be easy to see from the desire not to spend the length of time involved in pursuing two degrees plus years in residency training. However, raised are additional questions of whether an oral surgeon without an MD degree will be welcomed equally compared to someone with both dental and MD doctorates, as it relates to obtaining hospital privileges, access to surgical time, and respect in the workforce and general community.

The second example raises the question of "Where does dental hygiene fit?". Interesting historic perspectives provided in **Box 4** are from the 1926 paper presented by Fones.[37] Barriers and attitudes toward women in the workforce, their promotion, progress, and respect have been consistent overtime. Many issues discussed today surrounding the relationship between the practice of dentistry and the role of the dental hygienist were discussed 100 years ago. Given the poor oral health status of many Americans, models for increasing prevention and access care continue to evolve with dental hygienists central to the role as preventive specialists. **Box 5** displays data on the range of dental programs that fall under accreditation via the Commission on Dental Accreditation.[38] Seeing the disproportionate number of programs located in two-year institutions versus dental schools provides insight into some of the difficulties around achieving inclusivity across the full field of dentistry. Traditionally, few areas of dentistry directly experience coeducation, such that much of the training would be in isolation from other components of dentistry and allied dental team members. Seen in the 2022 to 2023 data, only 24 dental schools have dental hygiene programs associated with their universities.[20,38] Only 7% of dental hygiene programs are in proximity to training within dental schools, leaving about a third (32%) of

---

Box 3
Historic review of inclusion in oral and maxillofacial surgery via dual-degree surgeons: the example of Harvard University[35,36]

In 1846, first public demonstration of ether anesthesia in surgery was conducted in Boston by dental surgeons William Morton and Nathan Colley Keep.

In 1867, first university-affiliated dental school Harvard University established, with Keep as its first dean after his seeking establishment of dental education as part of medical education was denied: "My own predilection would favor a thorough and united dental and medical education."

In 1971, Harvard University Medical School approved awarding oral maxillofacial surgeons an MD degree with creation of a dual-degree program with Harvard School of Dental Medicine dental graduates as they had been in the same basic science training as the medical students.

In 1985, Harvard Medical School approved acceptance of non-Harvard School of Dental Medicine dental students into the dual-doctoral program with an additional year of training and two years of medical school.

In 1995, the Harvard Dual Doctoral program changed to all residents, regardless of where they attended dental school, in a 6- year program with 2 years of medical school.

Box 4
Brief history of the development of dental hygiene in the United States[37]

In 1844, the American Journal of Dental Science Editorial "Dental Hygiene" calling for more attention to the hygiene of the teeth.

1870 McLain A paper on "Prophylaxis or the Prevention of Dental Decay"

1879 First record of "cleaning of the teeth as carried out by the dentist."

1884 Rhein ML article "Oral Hygiene" recommended dentists teach their patients to brush their teeth effectively.

1884 Kingsley NW article "Women – Her position in dentistry" that advocated for women as assistants to the dentists and with experience "she will perform all operations required upon deciduous teeth, including fillings with any of the plastics ...."

1902 Wright CM presentation at the Odontological Society in Cincinnati "A Plea for a Sub-specialty in Dentistry" to be "women of education and refinement", provided education containing "special clinical training in prophylactic therapeutics," for positions "just as physicians and surgeons recommend and insist upon the services of the trained nurse ...."

1902 Low FW suggested the "Odontocure—a girl with an orange wood stick, some pumice, and possibly a flannel rag, who shall go from house to house ... with polishing teeth every 2 weeks ... possibly 50 cents would be the charge."

1903 Rhein ML proposed "The Dental Nurse" to the Section on Stomatology of the American Medical Association.

1906 Dr Fones had his office assistant, Mrs Irene Newman begin "prophylactic work for the patients... as far as we know was the first lay woman to practice dental prophylaxis."

1907 "The Connecticut dental law was amended to make it unlawful for dentists to employ unlicensed assistants for operative work in their offices" albeit further amended to allow for "so-called operation of cleaning teeth."

~1911, "The name 'dental hygienist' generally accepted."

1915 "Amendment of the Connecticut dental law ... legally prescribed for the first time the field of operation of the dental hygienist."

1916 "First university course [a full academic year in length] for dental hygienists ... now conducted by the College of Dentistry of Columbia University."

In 1923, the American Dental Hygienists' Association formed ... sponsored by the American Dental Association

---

dental schools with dental hygiene programs. This dynamic has helped to create a co-educational gap that has been difficult to close even with implementation of programming to deliberately promote collaborative practices such as interprofessional education (IPE).

A third example asks "What responsibilities and actions have dentistry and other health care professions had that helped to integrate versus separate the professions?" **Box 6** provides a brief layout of the history of health care integration and separation with a consideration of the influence of the event.[33,39–50] Decisive points happened along the history of dentistry and US health care that yielded notable inclusion and exclusion of dentistry. Some examples happened with dentistry's leadership making deliberate choices and others appeared to have happened with dentistry not being included at the decision-making table. An important lesson to dentistry is to get to the "table" and work to remain there to contribute toward identifying viable solutions to address the oral health crisis in our communities.

Box 5
US Commission on Dental Accreditation (CODA) Standards exist for these dental education programs and the corresponding number of recognized programs[38]

Allied Dental Education Programs = 582 (All in the United States)

Dental Assisting = 226	Dental Hygiene = 340
Dental Laboratory Technology = 13	Dental Therapy = 3

Predoctoral (DDS/DMD) Dental Education Programs = 75

United States = 73	Outside United States = 2
	Saudi Arabia = 1 Turkey = 1

Advanced Dental Education Programs = 776 (All in the United States)

Advanced Education in General Dentistry = 95	Dental Anesthesiology = 9
Dental Public Health = 15	Endodontics = 56
General Practice Residency = 168	Oral and Maxillofacial Pathology = 15
Oral and Maxillofacial Radiology = 9	Oral and Maxillofacial Surgery = 101
Oral Medicine = 6	Orofacial Pain = 13
Orthodontics Total = 70	Pediatric Dentistry = 87
Periodontics = 57	Prosthodontics Total = 57

CHALLENGES WITH INCLUSION AND INTEGRATION FOR DENTISTRY AND MEDICINE

US health care coverage via insurance added to the divide between medicine and dentistry based on different responses at the onset of health insurance and managed care in the US. Dentistry was excluded at critical points, albeit by self-omission; examples are found in the comprehensive establishment of Medicaid and Medicare.[51–53] The recognition of both medicine and dentistry in health care and other professional activities varies across circumstances. However, at this point, factors potentially involved in disabling inclusion are evident. The 2003 Institute of Medicine (IOM) report on Unequal Treatment does mention dentistry or dental, but in the context of a service that may be included, not as a full partner.[54] The report[55] identifies an oral health-specific initiative of the Health Resources and Services Administration (HRSA[55]) to provide equitable health care to the nation's highest need communities, and the Health Care Financing Administration (HCFA). HCFA was created in 1977 to combine under one administration the oversight of the Medicare program, the Federal portion of the Medicaid program, and related quality assurance activities. HCFA was renamed the Centers for Medicare and Medicaid Services in July, 2001,[56] which preceded the 2014 HRSA "Integration of Oral Health and Primary Care Practice" initiative.[57] While Medicaid does cover oral health, the extent and type of coverage are determined by each respective state.[44] This limited inclusion is contrasted with Medicare that until recently has provided minimal coverage for dental structures or procedures.[44] These programs have shown a duality of providing some with access to oral health care, while for others reinforcement the imagery of the mouth outside the overall realm of health.

Interest in seeing oral health inclusion with integration into primary care is wide reaching. The Association of State and Territorial Dental Directors (ASTDD) is one example of an association that while not directly providing health care services, does participate in policy development emphasizing the importance of the Integration of Oral Health into Primary Care as seen in their recent ASTDD Policy statement of that name.[58] Their role in recognizing the need for integration is particularly valuable as their role in states can influence allocation of resources as advisors to their respective state's chief health officer as an affiliate of the Association of State and Territorial Health Officers.[59]

Box 6	
A brief history of health care integration and separation actions	
	Inclusive Direction
~1650 first Yiddish Medical Self-help book includes dental conditions[39]	+
1745 Separation of Surgeons and Barbers in London[40]	-
1765 first Medical school in what will be the United States[33]	-
1821 first Pharmacy school in the United States[33]	-
1840 first Dental college in the United States/World[33]	-
1869 first University based dental school in the United States[41]	+
1881 AMA Section on Stomatology founded[42]	+
1892 first Osteopathy school in the United States[33]	-
1925 AMA Section on Stomatology disbanded[42]	-
1926 Gies Report[42]	~
1947 first American Dental Association Specialty of Oral Surgery[41]	~
1948 NIDR opened as third Institute of NIH[43]	+
1965 Medicaid[44]	~
1965 Medicare[44]	-
2009 first Meeting of Interprofessional Education Consortium[45]	+
2014 HRSA Integration of Oral health and Primary Care Practice[46]	+
2015 Propose HEENT examination to be HEENOT[47]	+
2016 "Precision Medicine Initiative"[48] [not being the "Precision Healthcare Initiative"]	-
2022 WHO Global Oral Health Status Report and Commentary in The Lancet	+

Abbreviations: HEENOT, head, ears, eyes, nose, oral cavity, throat; HEENT, head, ears, eyes nose throat; AMA, American Medical Association

CREATING INCLUSIVE ENVIRONMENTS THROUGH RESEARCH AND PROGRAM FUNDING

Other ways of expanding inclusion have been from health research perspectives with the National Institutes of Health (NIH). The National Institute of Dental and Craniofacial Research (NIDCR), which was at its origin the National Institute of Dental Research, was founded in 1948.[43] NIH has developed cross-institute collaborations, which has been seen in such manners as co-release of grant mechanism announcements. For NIDCR, these collaborations seem especially productive with the National Cancer Institute, Maternal and Child Health Institute, and the National Institute on Minority Health and Health Disparities. NIH has other cross-cutting units that intersect with dentistry, such as the NIH Office of Research on Women's Health (ORWH). While the ORWH has demonstrated appreciation of dentistry and oral health, several recent reports have not been so strong in the inclusion of dentistry. An example being the 2024 collaboration between the ORWH and the National Academies of Science, Engineering, and Medicine on "Advancing Research on Chronic Conditions in Women,"[60] where representation of dentistry and oral health is missing.

The federal government has supported health care provider training for development of a primary care workforce to correspond the growth of the US population through several significant programs. The first phases of these types of programs included medicine and dentistry. Programs such as Health Careers Opportunity Grants provided significant funding the support these initiatives[61] but then shifted to solely medicine.[62] Integration is being sought again, including debate over the professional degree for dentistry.[63,64] An overview of federal activities aimed at the integration of dentistry and medicine was provided in 2016.[65]

> **Box 7**
> **DEIB definitions within the framework of the American Dental Education Association[66]**
>
> 1. *Diversity*: Recognizes that each individual is unique with multiple dimensions of diversity that intersect, whether seen or unseen, and that society and community life benefit from the engagement of these differences regardless of culture, values, beliefs, race, ethnicity, language, age, sex, gender identity, sexual orientation, nationality, military/veteran status, disabilities, religion, economic status, geography, or other characteristics or ideologies.
>
> 2. *Equity*: The fair treatment, access, opportunity, and advancement for all people, while at the same time striving to identify and eliminate barriers that have prevented the full participation of some groups. The principle of equity acknowledges that there are historically underserved and underrepresented populations and that fairness regarding these unbalanced conditions is needed to assist in the provision of adequate opportunities to all groups.
>
> 3. *Inclusion*: The practice of leveraging diversity to ensure individuals can fully participate and perform at their best. Inclusion is shared responsibility of everyone within the community. An inclusive environment values differences rather than suppressing them; promotes respect, success, and a sense of belonging; and fosters well-being through policies, programs, practices, learning, and dialogue.
>
> 4. *Belonging*: The extent to which a person feels connected to or a part of the campus community and includes one's subjective evaluation of the quality of connections with others on campus or in the community. A sense of belonging contains both cognitive and affective aspects of the individual's cognitive assessment of their role in relationship to the group. Factors that may impact belongingness for historically underrepresented and marginalized groups include interactions with diverse peers, campus engagement in activities, the view of the overall climate, and exposure to bias, harassing, or discriminatory treatment.
>
> *Definition of Diversity, Inclusion & Belonging: Smith SG, Lee A, Gilbert JM. ADEA Faculty Diversity Toolkit, Appendix B—Diversity and Inclusion Terminology. Washington, DC: American Dental Education Association, 2020, pp. 164, 168, 172. At: https://www.adea.org/diversitytoolkit/, accessed August 1, 2024. **Definition of Equity: University of California, Davis. (2017). Diversity and Inclusion Strategic Vision. UC Davis: Diversity, Equity, and Inclusion. Retrieved from https://escholarship.org/uc/item/19s3j6h2

INCLUSIVITY IN HEALTH PROFESSIONS EDUCATION
The American Dental Education Association

The American Dental Education Association (ADEA) Strategic Directions 2019 to 2022 Workgroup spearheaded by Dr. Karen West (President, CEO of the ADEA, 2022) *"stressed the importance of developing and sustaining inclusive environments in which faculty, students, staff, and administrators work together to create the future of dental education in an increasingly diverse and interconnected world … not only assists dental education in recruiting and retaining a more diverse faculty but also moves academic dentistry forward in its pursuit of inclusive excellence."*[66] **Box 7** defines the components of the DEIB concept of ADEA.

The Interprofessional Education Collaborative

The founding of the Interprofessional Education Collaborative (IPEC)[67] provided a means for involving dentistry in IPE and collaborative practice. In a recent article, authors indicate that the IPE core competencies are important in elevating education and care, but the mark is missed if equity is not part of the discussion.[68] Additionally, the

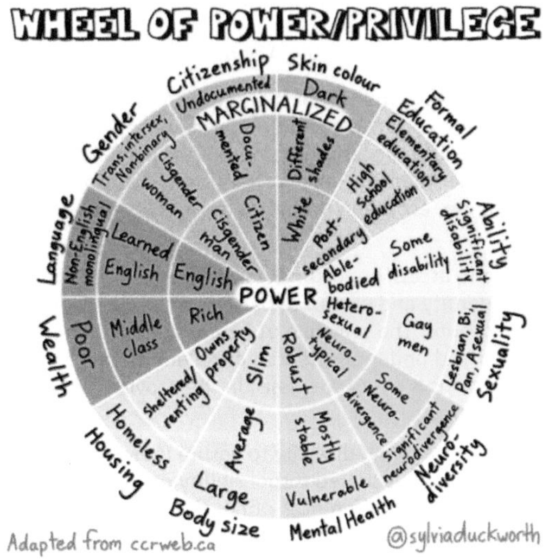

Fig. 2. An intersectionality wheel with emphasis on power and privilege structures.[76] (Duckworth S. Wheel of Power and Privilege. Wheel of Power, Privilege, and Marginalization, by Sylvia Duckworth. https://sdpride.org/wp-content/uploads/2022/11/Wheelof-Power-Privilege-Sylvia-Duckworth.pdf.)

observation is made that inclusion of dentistry is not conveyed in recent reports on outcomes assessment of IPE done in conjunction with IPEC.[69,70] This oversight further demonstrates the need to engage externally across the professions as well as internally within dentistry to continue to explore ways to expand efforts to promote and achieve inclusion with the dental profession.

The Importance of Intersectionality to Inclusion

In trying to make topics simple and easy to address, important information can be lost. The evolution of intersectionality seeks to provide useful and actionable information for addressing inequalities and operationalizing inclusion in the complex world. The concepts are not unlike mediation and confounding of epidemiology but argue for identifying and naming elements for transparently telling the story. Initial work in and attention to intersectionality stems from Sojourner Truth and her 1851 speech "Ain't I a Woman,"[71] Kimberle Crenshaw's introduction of the term in 1989 legal scholarship,[72] and the frequently cited 2012 work of Lisa Bowleg.[73] An example of application of these basic concepts to dentistry is presented in the Fleming and colleagues 2022 paper[74] where the increasing representation of women in dentistry in the United States and the United Kingdom "was not equal across all racial/ethnic groups. The largest increase in the number of female dentists was among White and Asian Women."[74]

While the focus of intersectionality originated with the consideration of Black Women, the breadth and depth of intersectionality have intensified. Factors to be recognized for their potential to add to inequalities and disparities follow those of social determinates of health,[75] as well as personal factors such as English proficiency, health/dental insurance coverage, religious practices, and gender identity. **Fig. 2** provides visual assistance for tracking the complexity of factors, including influence and power, in intersectionality.[76]

MOVING FURTHER ON INCLUSION IN DENTISTRY

The discussion presented earlier advocates that dentistry should be encouraged to craft criteria that exemplify, enable, and engage inclusive patient-centered health care practices and environments that are tailored for the levels of the profession across educational institutions, individual providers, and workspaces, as well as into the community. Such is the bedrock as the foundation for supporting the further building of diversity, equity, intersectionality, language, gender, culture, and ableism skills for optimizing the practice of dentistry.

CLINICS CARE POINTS

- Dentistry continues to evolve with an inclusive environment welcoming to all helping with problem-solving and optimizing oral health for all.
- Dentistry must be seated at the health care discussion and decision-making tables with the recognition of the bidirectionality needed for sustaining inclusion of oral health in general health.
- Dental education and practice need to recognize the nuances of multiple identities that people have and bring to consideration for developing inclusive, welcoming, and engaging environments.
- The dental profession must maintain momentum in promoting an inclusive environment that celebrates the oral health care team and remains collaborative as well as part of the solution to eliminating oral health disparities and inequalities.

DISCLOSURE

The authors have nothing to disclose.

REFERENCES

1. American Dental Association. The changing face of dentistry — meeting the challenge a diversity and inclusion toolkit for state and local dental societies. 2021. Available at: https://www.ada.org/-/media/project/ada-organization/ada/ada-org/files/membership/dental-societies/ada_diversity_inclusion_toolkit_2021. Accessed July 31, 2024.
2. American Dental Education Association. ADEA access, diversity and inclusion strategic framework 1-1. 2018. Available at: https://www.adea.org/diversity/framework/. Accessed May 20, 2024.
3. FDI World Dental Federation. National health policy. 2018. Available at: https://www.fdiworlddental.org/sites/default/files/2020-11/fdi_world_dental_federation_-_national_health_policy_-_2018-11-12.pdf. Accessed July 26, 2024.
4. FDI World Dental Federation. Our Purpose (no date), Available at: https://www.fdiworlddental.org/our-purpose. (Accessed 26 July 2024).
5. International Association for Dental Research. Science policy: diversity, equity, inclusion, accessibility, and belonging statement. (undated). Available at: https://www.iadr.org/science-policy/diversity-equity-inclusion-accessibility-and-belonging-statement. Accessed July 26, 2024.
6. National Academies of Sciences, Engineering, and Medicine. Ending unequal treatment: Strategies to achieve equitable health care and optimal health for all. Washington, DC: The National Academies Press; 2024. p. 325. Available at: https://nap.nationalacademies.org/catalog/27820/ending-unequal-treatment-strategies-to-achieve-equitable-health-care-and. Accessed July 31, 2024.

7. White house Executive Order (14035) on diversity, equity, inclusion, and accessibility in the federal workforce, Available at: https://www.whitehouse.gov/briefing-room/presidential-actions/2021/06/25/executive-order-on-diversity-equity-inclusion-and-accessibility-in-the-federal-workforce/ (Accessed 29 July 2024), 2021.
8. Vespa J, Median L, Armstrong DM. Demographic turning points for the United States: population projections for 2020 to 2060. Current Population Reports. Washington, DC: US Census Bureau; 2020. p. 25–1144. Available at: https://www.census.gov/content/dam/Census/library/publications/2020/demo/p25-1144.pdf. Accessed July 31, 2024.
9. Mason BS, Heath C, Parker J, et al. Diversity, equity, inclusion and belonging in dermatology. Dermatol Clin 2023;41(2):239–48.
10. Sinkford JC, Smith SG. Introduction to this special issue. J Dent Educ 2022;86:1051–4.
11. Anderson TH. The pursuit of fairness: a history of affirmative action. New York: Oxford University Press; 2004.
12. The Constitution of the United States: a transcript. Available at: https://www.archives.gov/founding-docs/constitution-transcript. Accessed July 26, 2024.
13. Zangwill I. The melting pot. 1908. Available at: https://www.pbs.org/fmc/timeline/emeltpot.htm. Accessed July 26, 2024.
14. Thornton BS. Melting pots and salad bowls: what is the future of assimilation in America? Hoover digest. Hoover institution. Washington, DC: Stanford University; 2012. Available at: https://www.hoover.org/research/melting-pots-and-salad-bowls. Accessed July 26, 2024.
15. Coan J. America: not a melting pot, not a salad bowl, but a chili bowl. New York: Braver Angels; 2020. Available at: https://braverangels.org/america-not-a-melting-pot-not-a-salad-bowl-but-a-chili-bowl/. Accessed July 26, 2024.
16. Setiloane KT. Beyond the melting pot and salad bowl views of cultural diversity: advancing cultural diversity education of nutrition educators. J Nutr Educ Behav 2016;48(9):664–8.e1.
17. DeLaRosa J. Melting pot or boiling pot? Exploring our society's diversity. Ann Thorac Surg 2022;114:18–9.
18. Ring M, Ai D, Maker-Clark G, et al. Cooking up change: DEIB principles as key ingredients in nutrition and culinary medicine education. Nutrients 2023;15(19):4257.
19. American dental association health policy institute. U.S. Dentists demographics dashboard. 2020. Available at: https://www.ada.org/resources/research/health-policy-institute/dentist-workforce. Accessed July 31, 2024.
20. American Dental Association Health Policy Institute. Dental education, Available at: https://www.ada.org/resources/research/health-policy-institute/dental-education. (Accessed 31 July 2024), 2020.
21. American Dental Education Association. Number of full-time and part-time dental school faculty by race and ethnicity, 2018-19 academic year, Available at: https://www.adea.org/data/Faculty/2018-2019-Survey/. (Accessed 29 May 2024).
22. Weinstein GJ, Haden NK, Stewart DCL, et al. A profile of dental school deans, 2021. J Dent Educ 2022;86(10):1304–16.
23. Bompolaki D, Pokala SV, Koka S. Gender diversity and senior leadership in academic dentistry: female representation at the dean position in the United States. J Dent Educ 2022;86(4):401–5.
24. The white house. Fact sheet: president biden signs executive order advancing diversity, equity, inclusion, and accessibility in the federal government. Available

at: https://www.whitehouse.gov/briefing-room/statements-releases/2021/06/25/fact-sheet-president-biden-signs-executive-order-advancing-diversity-equity-inclusion-and-accessibility-in-the-federal-government/. Accessed August 1, 2024.

25. Norbash A, Kadom N. The business case for diversity and inclusion. J Am Coll Radiol 2020;17(5):676–80.
26. Frei F, Morriss A. Move fast and fix things: the trusted leader's guide to solving hard problems. Boston: Harvard Business Review Press; 2023.
27. Wei W, Cai Z, Ding J, et al. Organizational leadership gender differences in medical schools and affiliated universities. J Womens Health (Larchmt) 2024;33(5): 662–70.
28. Koop CE. Paper presented at Oral Health 2000, Second National Consortium Advance Program. 1993.
29. Allukian M Jr. The neglected epidemic and the surgeon general's report: a call to action for better oral health. Am J Publ Health 2008;98(9 Suppl):S82–5.
30. Oral Health in America: Advances and Challenges, Bethesda (MD): National Institute of Dental and Craniofacial Research (US) Section 1: Effect of oral health on the community, overall well-being, and the economy, 2021, Available at: https://www.ncbi.nlm.nih.gov/books/NBK578297/. (Accessed 29 July 2024).
31. In appreciation of Dr. C. Everett Koop quotes with image, Available at: https://www.bookey.app/quote-author/c-everett-koop. (Accessed 30 July 2024).
32. Borkman T., In appreciation of Dr. C. Everett Koop, *Int'l J self-help self-care*, 5 (4), 2006-2007, 299–305, Available at: https://triggered.stanford.clockss.org/ServeContent?url=http%3A%2F%2Fbaywood.stanford.clockss.org%2FBWSH%2FBAWOOD_BWSH_5_4%2FHH465492847T82G6.pdf. (Accessed 30 July 2024).
33. Kaste LM, Halpern LR. The barber pole might have been an early sign for patient-centered care: what do interprofessional education and interprofessional collaborative practice look like now? Dent Clin North Am 2016;60(4):765–88.
34. Chaudhary PP, Kaur M, Myles IA. Does "all disease begin in the gut"? The gut-organ cross talk in the microbiome. Appl Microbiol Biotechnol 2024;108(1):339.
35. Kaban LB, Perrott DH. Dual-degree oral and maxillofacial surgery training in the United States: "Back to the Future". J Oral Maxillofac Surg 2020;78:18–28.
36. Kaban LB, Hale R, Perrott DH. Oral and maxillofacial surgery training in the United States: influences of dental and medical education, wartime experiences, and other external factors. Oral Maxillofac Surg Clin 2022;495–503.
37. Fones AC. The origin and history of the dental hygienist movement. JADA (J Am Dent Assoc) 1926;13(12):1809–21.
38. CODA the Commission on Dental Accreditation. Find a program, Available at: https://coda.ada.org/. (Accessed 31 July 2024).
39. Ring ME. Dental writings in a medical self-help book of 1650. J Hist Dent 2004; 52(3):125–9.
40. Wynbrandt J. The excruciating history of dentistry: toothsome tales & oral oddities from Babylon to Braces. New York: St Martin's Griffin; 1998.
41. American Dental Association. 150 Years of the American Dental Associaiton: a pictorial history, 1859-2009. Chicago: American Dental Association; 2009.
42. Gies W.J., Dental education in the United States and Canada: A report to the Carnegie Foundation for the Advancement of Teaching, 1926, The Carnegie Foundation for the Advancement of Teaching; New York, Available at: https://www.adea.org/ADEAGiesFoundation/William-J-Gies-and-Gies-Report.aspx. (Accessed 1 August 2024).
43. Sheridan PG. NIDR–40 years of research advances in dental health. Publ Health Rep 1988;103(5):493–9.

44. Centers for Medicare and Medicaid Services. CMS program history Medicare and Medicaid, Available at: https://www.cms.gov/about-cms/who-we-are/history. (Accessed 1 August 2024).

45. Interprofessional Education Collaborative Expert Panel. Core competencies for interprofessional collaborative practice: report of an expert panel. Washington, DC: Interprofessional Education Collaborative; 2011.

46. Health Resources and Services Administration. Integration of oral health and primary care practice. Rockville (MD): US Department of Health and Human Services Health Resources and services Administration; 2014. Available at: https://www.hrsa.gov/sites/default/files/hrsa/oral-health/integration-oral-health.pdf. Accessed August 1, 2024.

47. Haber J, Hartnett E, Allen K, et al. Putting the mouth back in the head: HEENT to HEENOT. Am J Publ Health 2015;105(3):437–41.

48. The Obama White House. The precision medicine initiative, Available at: https://obamawhitehouse.archives.gov/precision-medicine. (Accessed 1 August 2024), 2016.

49. World Health Organization. Global oral health status report: towards universal health coverage for oral health by 2030. Geneva (Switzerland): World Health Organization; 2022.

50. Benzian H, Watt R, Makino Y, et al. WHO calls to end the global crisis of oral health. Lancet 2022;400(10367):1909–10.

51. Simon L. Overcoming historical separation between oral and general health care: interprofessional collaboration for promoting health equity. AMA J Ethics 2016; 18(9):941–9.

52. Mertz EA. The dental-medical divide. Health Aff 2016;35(12):2168–75.

53. Braunold J. Why don't medicare and medicaid cover dental health services? AMA J Ethics 2022;24(1):E89–98.

54. Institute of Medicine. Unequal treatment: confronting racial and ethnic disparities in health care. Washington, DC: The National Academies Press; 2003.

55. Health resources and services administration. Home. Who we are. Available at: https://www.hrsa.gov/. Accessed August 1, 2024.

56. Centers for Medicare & Medicaid Services. Home. What are you looking for today?. Available at: https://www.cms.gov/. Accessed August 1, 2024.

57. US Department of Health and Human Services Health Resources and Services Administration. Integration of oral health and primary care practice, Available at: https://www.hrsa.gov/sites/default/files/hrsa/oral-health/integration-oral-health.pdf. (Accessed 1 August 2024), 2014.

58. Association of State and Territorial Dental Directors. Policy statement: integrating oral health care into primary care, Available at: https://www.astdd.org/docs/integrating-oral-health-care-into-primary-care.pdf. (Accessed 1 August 2024).

59. Association od State and Territorial Health Officials. ASTHO Councils, Available at: https://www.astho.org/about/governance/astho-councils/. (Accessed 1 August 2024).

60. National Academies of Sciences, Engineering, and Medicine. Advancing research on chronic conditions in women. Washington, DC: The National Academies Press; 2024.

61. Reynolds PP. A legislative history of federal assistance for health professions training in primary care medicine and dentistry in the United States, 1963-2008. Acad Med 2008;83(11):1004–14.

62. Phillips RL Jr, Turner BJ. The next phase of Title VII funding for training primary care physicians for America's health care needs. Ann Fam Med 2012;10(2): 163–8.
63. Giddon DB, Lamster IB. The dilemma of different dental degrees: DDS and DMD. J Dent Educ 2022;86(8):998–1005.
64. Atchison KA, Rozier RG, Weintraub JA. Integration of oral health and primary care: communication, coordination, and referral. NAM Perspectives. Discussion Paper. Washington, DC: National Academy of Medicine; 2018.
65. Joskow CR. Integrating oral health and primary care: federal initiatives to drive systems change. Dent Clin North Am 2016;60(4):951–68.
66. Smith SG, Lee A, Gilbert JM. ADEA faculty diversity toolkit. Available at: https://www.adea.org/diversitytoolkit/. Accessed August 1, 2024.
67. Interprofessional Education Collaborative (IPEC), Available at: https://www.ipecollaborative.org/. (Accessed 1 August 2024).
68. Prelock PA, Johnson AF. Advancing IPE and equity in complex systems of care. ASHA Journals Academy. Available at: https://academy.pubs.asha.org/2021/12/advancing-ipe-and-equity-in-complex-systems-of-care/. Accessed August 1, 2024.
69. Cadet T, Cusimano J, McKearney S, et al. Describing the evidence linking interprofessional education interventions to improving the delivery of safe and effective patient care: a scoping review. J Interprof Care 2024;38(3):476–85.
70. Reeves S, Perrier L, Goldman J, et al. Interprofessional education: effects on professional practice and healthcare outcomes (update). Cochrane Database Syst Rev 2013;2013(3):CD002213.
71. Truth S. "Ain't I A woman?" Delivered at the 1851 Women's Convention, Akron, Ohio. Available at: https://tag.rutgers.edu/wp-content/uploads/2014/05/Aint-I-woman.pdf. Accessed August 1, 2024 https://www.commonlit.org/en/texts/ain-t-i-a-woman-1.
72. Crenshaw KW. Demarginalizing the intersection of race and sex. A Black feminist critique of antidiscrimination doctrine, Feminist Theory and Antiracist Politics. 1989; Iss. 1: University of Chicago Legal Forum. Article 8. Available at: http://chicagounbound.uchicago.edu/uclf/vol1989/iss1/8. Accessed July 29, 2024.
73. Bowleg L. The problem with the phrase women and minorities: intersectionality-an important theoretical framework for public health. Am J Publ Health 2012; 102(7):1267–73.
74. Fleming E, Neville P, Muirhead VE. Are there more women in the dentist workforce? Using an intersectionality lens to explore the feminization of the dentist workforce in the UK and US. Community Dent Oral Epidemiol 2023;51(3):365–72.
75. Watt RG, Mathur MR, Aida J, et al. Oral health disparities in children: a canary in the coalmine? Pediatr Clin North Am 2018;65(5):965–79.
76. Duckworth S. Wheel of power and privilege. Available at: https://sdpride.org/wp-content/uploads/2022/11/Wheel-of-Power-Privilege-Sylvia-Duckworth.pdf. Accessed August 1, 2024 https://www.instagram.com/p/CEHUShhpUT/?hl=en https://www.researchgate.net/publication/364109273_Migrants_at_the_university_doorstep_How_we_unfairly_deny_access_and_what_we_could_should_do_now/figures?lo=1 https://www.thisishowyoucan.com/post/__wheel_of_power_and_privilege https://www.instagram.com/sylviaduckworth/ https://sylviaduckworth.com/.

Inclusive Language to Support Health Equity and Belonging in Dentistry

Colin M. Haley, DDS, MEd, MHA[a],*, Alison F. Doubleday, MA, MS, PhD[b]

KEYWORDS

- Inclusive language • Health equity • Belonging • Person-centered care • Diversity
- Inclusion • Dentistry

KEY POINTS

- Inclusive language in dentistry is crucial for creating a respectful, empathetic environment that acknowledges and supports patients from diverse backgrounds, promoting health equity and a sense of belonging.
- Inclusive language involves using respectful, accurate, unbiased language, focusing on person-first language, and being aware of the evolving nature of language to reflect individuals' preferences and community standards.
- Language is embedded in health care systems and can reinforce or challenge biases.
- Education and training in inclusive language for all oral health care providers and staff are essential to integrate the principles of health equity and belonging in practice, improve patient–provider relationships, and enhance health care outcomes.

INTRODUCTION

Oral health care providers are entrusted with the care of patients from a vast array of backgrounds, each with their unique needs, experiences, and expectations. Caring for diverse patients, many that have been historically excluded from receiving equitable care, requires us to actively acquire new knowledge that is aligned with inclusive, person-centered care principles. This approach ensures care that is customized to each individual's identities, beliefs, and needs.[1] Inclusive care stands on the principle that everyone deserves high-quality health care that is respectful, empathetic, and meets their unique needs, regardless of their background or identity.

In health care, including the dental clinic setting, establishing trust is crucial for successful relationships, and adopting person-centered care principles fosters this trust.[2]

[a] Department of Oral Medicine and Diagnostic Sciences, College of Dentistry, University of Illinois Chicago, 801 S. Paulina Street, Room 204C, Chicago, IL 60612, USA; [b] Department of Oral Medicine and Diagnostic Sciences, College of Dentistry, University of Illinois Chicago, 801 S. Paulina Street, Room 527, Chicago, IL 60612, USA
* Corresponding author.
E-mail address: Chaley1@uic.edu

Dent Clin N Am 69 (2025) 17–28
https://doi.org/10.1016/j.cden.2024.08.001
0011-8532/25/© 2024 Elsevier Inc. All rights are reserved, including those for text and data mining, AI training, and similar technologies.
dental.theclinics.com

The role of language is a critical tool in fulfilling the promise of trusting and inclusive care, acting not just as a means to convey information, but also as a way to express respect, empathy, and understanding. Employing inclusive language is vital for creating an environment where patients of all backgrounds feel acknowledged and understood, underscoring the importance of language in effectively delivering inclusive care.

While inclusive language is broadly defined as language that avoids certain words or expressions that might exclude particular groups of people, it is widely accepted that inclusive language must go beyond exclusion. Inclusive language should be "respectful, accurate, unbiased, and consistent with the preferences of the individuals and communities who are discussed."[3] Using inclusive language in our health care practices and educational settings supports our patients, staff, and students in a manner that reinforces both health equity, which is the state in which everyone has a fair and just opportunity to attain their highest level of health, and belonging, or the sense of security and support when there is a sense of acceptance and inclusion.[4] Adopting inclusive language within the oral health care setting is an essential step toward integrating the principles of health equity and belonging into everything oral health care providers do. Through the use of inclusive language, every individual can feel seen, heard, and valued, all while moving toward a more equitable oral health care system.

Inclusive language should be utilized in all contexts and is equally important in the clinical setting between providers and patients, among providers and staff, and in the educational setting, as a way to support student development and to model best practices. As we move forward in our discussion, it is important to note the distinction between language and communication. Language is the structured system of symbols, words, and rules we use to convey messages, while communication encompasses the broader process of exchanging information, thoughts, and feelings through various means, including language, gestures, and other nonverbal cues. Communication encompasses shared terminology (language) as well as narrative and nonverbal means of representing thoughts, emotions, and ideas.[5] In a clinical setting, the importance of language between providers and patients acts as the cornerstone for building trust and understanding. Inclusive language facilitates clear communication and reduces misunderstandings and misinterpretations that can lead to misdiagnosis, dissatisfaction, or inadequate treatment.[6] By acknowledging each patient's unique identity, health care providers can create a welcoming and safe environment that encourages patients to share vital information about their health, lifestyle, and concerns, leading to more accurate assessments and personalized care plans.[7]

Among providers and staff, the adoption of inclusive language fosters a culture of respect, acknowledging and valuing diversity while improving an individual's sense of belonging. Inclusive language in the workplace has additional benefits including reducing discrimination and bias, improving communication and collaboration, and building trust and respect.[8] Benefits such as improving communication and collaboration can improve job efficacy, support retention of clinical staff, reduce adverse clinical events and outcomes, and are among the most important factors in improving clinical effectiveness and job satisfaction.[9]

Within the educational setting, language has profound effects and influences learners' feelings of belonging, resilience, identity, self-efficacy, and achievement.[10] Language acts as a mirror, reflecting the values and norms of the educational setting, and thereby shaping the professional identity of future health care providers. Lapses in shared understanding due to non-inclusive language risk alienating learners, patients, and colleagues create barriers to effective communication and empathy.[11] Modeling inclusive language is paramount for educators, as it equips future health care providers with the necessary skills to engage with patients from diverse backgrounds in a respectful and understanding manner. Through deliberate practice and emphasis on inclusive language, health professions educators can ensure that the next generation of providers is not only clinically competent, but also culturally responsive and inclusive in their practice.

DISCUSSION: INCLUSIVE LANGUAGE IN THE CLINICAL SETTING

In the health care setting, the adoption of inclusive language is essential for fostering a respectful environment that values each patient's unique background and needs. Inclusive language is characterized by its nonjudgmental nature, reliance on facts, and the practice of mentioning personal characteristics only when they are medically relevant.[12] This approach avoids stigmatization and ensures that communication does not inadvertently harm or alienate patients. By focusing on facts and relevance, health care providers can create a more welcoming and supportive space for all patients. Using inclusive language in practice requires an understanding of general guidelines, key principles, and community-specific preferences.

General Guidelines

1. *Use plain language*: Plain language is a straightforward way of communicating that avoids complex vocabulary, making information accessible to people of all reading levels and backgrounds. This simplicity ensures that important health information is not obscured by medical jargon, which can often be intimidating or misunderstood by patients. It is equally important to avoid use of expressions or idioms that may not translate well across different cultures or may carry unintended connotations.[13]
2. *Listen*: Listening is a cornerstone of inclusive communication. Providers should actively listen to patients, giving them space to share if something is harmful or uncomfortable for them. This space for open dialogue can reveal when certain terms or phrases may be distressing or inappropriate, allowing for immediate correction and education. Listening is an essential skill for effective communication between individuals of different backgrounds and with diverse life experiences.[14]
3. *Set aside assumptions*: Implicit bias and the use of associated stigmatizing language have far-reaching effects, automatically activating stereotypes that can influence judgments and behaviors in subtle, often unrecognized ways.[15] Health care providers must not presume to know the experiences or needs of their patients based on their appearance, background, or health condition. Setting aside assumptions and being aware of our own biases avoid stereotyping and also open the door for patients to share their unique perspectives and needs in an open way.
4. *Consider context*: Understand historical contexts of language as words are often rooted in oppression. Certain terms that were once widely used may carry a history of derogatory or exclusionary use (such as blacklist or blackmail, which may associate the color black with negative or bad characteristics). Educating oneself about these historical contexts is key to understanding why some terms should be avoided. Inclusive language may also be context dependent, with a word or phrase being appropriate in one context while being considered harmful in another, thus emphasizing the need to understand the preference of individuals and communities.[16]
5. *Always evolving*: Language is not static; it is always evolving. As society becomes more aware of the experiences of individuals and groups, language adapts to reflect this awareness. Health care providers must stay informed about these changes and the reasons behind them to remain respectful and relevant in their interactions with others. Communities and individuals may also change their

preferences overtime, and it is important to understand when preferred language shifts.[3]

6. *Be aware of preferred terms*: While there are overarching guidelines that providers can follow, the preference for terms and language is determined by the individual and community. A discussion of current preferences of some communities is discussed later in this article.

7. *Should be utilized everywhere*: Inclusive language is not limited to a single setting and is applicable from the waiting area to the clinical room. Training on the use of inclusive language should occur for all individuals who work in the oral health setting, the principles of which can be utilized in all settings in the health care environment.

Key Principles

Person-first language

The role of person-first language in fostering an inclusive clinical environment is integral to delivering compassionate and respectful care. Person-first language places the individual before any characteristic or diagnosis they might have, humanizing the individual and avoiding reduction to a single aspect of their identity. By emphasizing the person rather than a particular condition, health care providers acknowledge the patient's value and identity beyond their health challenges.

The importance of person-first language lies in its ability to reshape perceptions. It counteracts the stigma often associated with medical conditions and disabilities, which can be perpetuated through language and avoids using labels or adjectives to define someone.[17] For example, instead of referring to someone as "diabetic," person-first language would suggest saying "person with diabetes." This subtle shift changes the focus from the disease to the individual, recognizing that the condition is only one attribute of the person's complex identity.

Person-first language also extends to discussions about lifestyle or social circumstances. Instead of labeling someone as "homeless," which defines them solely by their lack of housing, it is more respectful to say "person experiencing homelessness" or "people without housing." This language implies a condition that is temporary and does not encompass the individual's entire identity.

The use of person-first language is not without its nuances. Some communities, particularly within the disability community, may prefer identity-first language, such as "autistic person" instead of "person with autism," as a way of embracing their disability as an integral part of their identity.[18] It is crucial for health care providers to ask individuals how they wish to be referred to and to honor their preferences. This dialogue reinforces the patient's autonomy and self-identification.

Avoid stigmatizing words

It is important to navigate away from terms that inadvertently stigmatize communities or individuals. Adjectives such as "vulnerable," "marginalized," and "high-risk" can carry implications that reinforce negative stereotypes or suggest inherent weakness or deficiency within groups or individuals. Instead, the focus should be on describing the structural and systemic factors that contribute to differing health outcomes among populations.

To avoid stigmatization, we can explain the broader context that leads to disparities. For instance, rather than labeling a community as "vulnerable," it may be more accurate and respectful to describe the specific conditions that contribute to their increased exposure to health risks, such as "communities with limited access to health care" or "populations affected by housing instability." This language acknowledges the external factors that contribute to health status without implying that the community's identity is the source of risk.[19]

Similarly, describing groups as "marginalized" can be replaced with explanations of the mechanisms of marginalization. For example, we can specify that "policies and social practices have historically limited this group's access to resources," thereby focusing on the actions that have led to their marginalization, rather than presenting marginalization as an attribute of the group itself.

Some common language used in health care unintentionally places blame on the individual such as labeling someone as "noncompliant" with their medications or treatment regimen. There are many reasons why an individual may be unable to adhere to recommendations, including finances, access, or social issues. Alternating the language to something like "unable to adhere due to ..." provides a clear description of the challenges the individual may be facing while not assigning blame to the patient.

It is also important to avoid language that has violent connotations. Patients come from many different backgrounds with a variety of personal experiences, some of which may be violent or traumatizing in nature. Some language may evoke negative responses from patients due to past trauma. Avoid language like "target, tackle, trigger" and replace them with alternatives such as "engage, prioritize, prompt" to provide a more neutral approach.[19]

Being aware of stigmatizing language in the clinical setting and choosing to use inclusive alternatives is important, not just in the personal interactions we have with patients, but also in the language we utilize in the written medical record. Inclusive language reinforces health equity as it is well documented that language that reinforces bias and stereotypes leads to negative attitudes toward patients and diminished health outcomes.[20] **Table 1** provides inclusive language alternatives to common words and phrases. **Table 2** demonstrates how small adjustments to wording, emphasizing neutral and person-first language, create a less stigmatizing patient encounter note.

Current Preferences

Language is fluid and dynamic, reflecting the ever-evolving landscape of cultural norms and societal values. What is deemed as preferred terminology today may shift in the future as we gain deeper understanding and as communities redefine the terms that best represent their identities. In the following list, we explore current preferred terminology and best practices in inclusive language across various domains:

1. *Race and ethnicity*: First, it is important to note the definitions of both race and ethnicity with race defined as "any one of the groups that humans are often divided into based on physical traits regarded as common among people of shared ancestry"[21] and ethnicity as "[t]he fact or state of belonging to a social group that has a shared national or cultural tradition."[22] Both terms can be identified as a social construct, and while their utility in understanding biology is limited, being critical about the way in which they contribute to racism and inequity is important. Preferred terminology around race and ethnicity emphasizes specificity and self-identification. It is best to use the terms that individuals use for themselves. Terms such as "Black" or "African American," "Hispanic," "Latino," or "Latina," "Asian," "Native American," or "Indigenous" should be capitalized to acknowledge their cultural significance. Avoid outdated terms or those with negative connotations. The general term "minorities" should be avoided when describing groups and populations because of the connotation that a community is less than or inferior. If racial and ethnic terms are used, they should not be used in noun form (Blacks, Whites,

Table 1
Inclusive language alternatives to common words and phrases

Rather than...	Use Instead
• Ladies and Gentlemen • You Guys	• Everyone • Colleagues • Y'all, you all
• Crazy • Insane	• Hectic • Chaotic
• Mother/father	• Parent • Guardian
• Husband/wife	• Spouse/partner
• Blacklist	• Allow list, deny list
• Vulnerable groups/marginalized groups • High risk	• Groups that have been marginalized or made vulnerable • Groups placed at increased risk due to ...
• Diabetic • Homeless	• Person living with diabetes • People who are experiencing homelessness or are unhoused
• Target communities • Tackle issues • Trigger	• Engage • Prioritize • Prompt
• Noncompliant	• Non-adherence/unable to adhere
• Minority/underrepresented	• Systematically excluded, under-recognized
• Addict	• Person with substance-use disorder

Hispanics, or Asians). If necessary for use, an adjectival form is preferred following American Medical Association (AMA) guidance regarding person-first language.[23]

2. *Diseases, disorders, and disabled*: The preferred approach in referring to diseases, disorders, and disabilities is person-first language, which acknowledges the person before the condition (eg, "person with epilepsy" rather than "epileptic"). As stated earlier, this is not a universal guideline with some groups, including some members of the autistic and deaf community, preferring identity-first language as they consider their condition an integral part of their identity. Some terms utilized in the past such as differently abled and handi-capable can often be viewed as condescending and reinforce the idea that someone living with a disability should be ashamed. These terms should be avoided unless preferred by an individual.[24] Additionally, some language labels individuals as victims and should also be

Table 2
Neutral, person-first, non-stigmatizing encounter note example

Encounter Note Excerpt	Encounter Note Excerpt: Inclusive Language Alternative
24 year old transgender patient presents for limited examination complaining of pain in upper right molar. Patient is a former heroin abuser, is HIV+, and has bipolar disorder. He has failed previous 3 dental visits and is homeless. He is currently noncompliant with medication regimen.	24 year old transgender patient (prefers they/them pronouns) presents for limited examination complaining of pain in upper right molar. They have a history of heroin substance use disorder and are currently living with HIV and bipolar disorder. Patient has been unable to make previous dental visits and maintain medication adherence due to being unhoused.

avoided. In each case, there are alternatives that emphasize the person not the disease, for example, saying "patient with diabetes" instead of "patient suffering from diabetes" or "person using a wheelchair" instead of "wheelchair bound." As always, it is important to ask and respect personal preferences.

3. *Age*: When addressing age, avoid patronizing or diminishing terms like "the elderly" or "the aged." Instead, use terms like "older adults" or "persons aged 65 years and older." Because "older" is a vague and relative term, the AMA Manual of Style recommends clinicians and researchers should state specific ages as appropriate.[25] For people younger than 18 years, "children" or "adolescents" are generally acceptable, but the specific age or developmental stage should be referenced if relevant to the care or context.[26]

4. *Socioeconomic status*: Discussions of socioeconomic status should be conducted with sensitivity and without judgment. Avoid stigmatizing terms like "poor" or "low class." Instead, use phrases like "persons of low socioeconomic status" or "individuals experiencing poverty." Recognize the complexity and diversity of experiences within this group and the systemic factors that contribute to socioeconomic status.[25,26]

5. *Sex, gender, and pronouns*: Language regarding sex and gender should be precise and respectful of individual identity. Distinguish between "sex," which refers to biological attributes, and "gender," which is a social identity of being male, female, or another gender identity. It is important to acknowledge the fluidity that occurs with both gender and sexual orientation (a personal pattern of attraction) as these can change overtime and can be nonbinary in nature.[27] Terms like "cisgender" (gender identity matches sex assigned at birth) and "transgender" (gender identity does not match sex assigned at birth) should be used appropriately. Avoid assumptions about gender based on names or appearances and refrain from using gendered language such as "ladies and gentlemen" in favor of gender-neutral alternatives like "everyone." In clinical settings, the use of gender-neutral language is a key strategy for inclusiveness. For example, replacing "mothers and fathers" with "parents" and "husbands and wives" with "spouses" or "partners" can avoid excluding non-heteronormative family structures.[17] When it comes to pronouns, always use the pronouns that the individual has specified. Using "they" as a singular form of gender-neutral pronoun is appropriate in all settings and avoids misgendering individuals that can cause distress and erode trust.[26] Modeling pronoun use in introductions to patients as well as providing inclusive intake forms can be helpful to allow individuals to share their own pronouns and validate their identity within the context of an inclusive clinical setting. Common lesbian, gay, bisexual, transgender, queer+ terminology and pronouns can be found in **Table 3**.

CHALLENGES
Structural Biases

Although the benefits and positive impact of the use of inclusive language in clinical education and in clinical encounters are widely acknowledged, there are significant challenges that must be addressed. Adopting inclusive language requires self-reflection and self-awareness, not just by individuals, but also by entire fields and professions. Structural racism and other biases are embedded within health professions processes and procedures. Organizational practices, in additional to individual biases, have the potential to sustain inequities for patients and trainees.[28] The language that is used within health care settings reflects these deep-rooted systems and can contribute to the perpetuation of structural biases. As a cultural tool, language shapes

Table 3	
Common lesbian, gay, bisexual, transgender, queer+ terms and pronouns	
LGBTQ+ Terminology	
LGBTQ+	Lesbian, gay, bisexual, transgender, queer and the + includes other members of the community.
Sex assigned at birth	The sex you were designated based on genitals and chromosomes (eg, male, female, or intersex).
Gender identity	The way in which someone perceives their own gender on a spectrum and which may or may not align with their sex assigned at birth (eg, cisgender woman, transgender or nonbinary, cisgender man).
Gender expression	How one performs their identity to society, however, you should not assume someone's identity based off of their gender expression (eg, feminine, androgynous, or nonbinary, masculine).
Sexual orientation	Refers to the way in which someone is attracted to others (eg, heterosexual, bisexual, pansexual, homosexual).
Pronouns	
Gender binary	She/her/hers He/him/his
Gender neutral	They/them/theirs Ze/hir/hirs Ze/zir/zirs Xe, xem, xyr

our expectations and behavior[29] and can subsequently reinforce biases and beliefs about stereotypes. An example of this is the use of medical jargon with a patient or use of complex medical terms in the early stages of a student's training, under the assumption that all preclinical students are familiar with medical terminology. When patients or students do not meet expectations for specific language comprehension, clinicians and educators may conclude that patients are problematic or non-adherent or that students are inattentive or incapable of being successful. When patients and students are part of systematically excluded groups, these conclusions can easily reinforce stereotypes or promote biases.[30] A better approach is to use clear and specific language with all patients and to intentionally develop vocabulary and discipline-specific terminology across all learners.[28] Health professionals may not always be aware of bias underpinning particular terminology or phrasing. Within educational settings, for example, language that is used to describe or define concepts like professionalism is often grounded in white, European standards for appearance and behavior and can be used to penalize systematically excluded or underrecognized students. For example, students or patients who take offense at or speak out against microaggressions may be labeled as "unprofessional." Biased language around success, progress, and professionalism in clinical education can interfere with a student's sense of belonging and can activate stereotype threat, the fear of confirming negative stereotypes associated with a particular group.[29] The resulting stress and anxiety stemming from these interactions can have a deleterious effect on academic and clinical performance, further reinforcing stereotypes or validating the language used. Rather than simply being a symptom of organizational and structural biases, the words and labels we use for categories "constitute a form of support in the creation and comprehension of the categories themselves."[29]

Language Barriers and Cultural Differences

Many patients find it necessary to use a second language to access health care services. Language discordant encounters in health care can lead to health communication anxiety as well as maintain health inequities.[31] Challenges associated with language proficiency and the need to use a second language in health care interactions include difficulty seeking information about available health services, as well as in interpreting health information and navigating the health care system, all resulting in associations between a patient's health status and their linguistic status, subsequently impacting emotional, mental, and physical health.[31] Cultural beliefs around oral health can also differ between patients and clinicians. These differences can contribute to a reluctance to seek health care and to communicate health care needs with clinicians as well. These differences can also contribute to the use of stigmatizing language by clinicians when referencing patient encounters as the beliefs that we have about people are reflected in our language. Recognizing the biases embedded in the language we use is not just important in our interpersonal interactions with patients and students but extends to the words we use to describe patients and learners to our colleagues, as well as to the stories we tell about the work we do. As mentioned previously, this is true regardless of whether stigmatizing language is communicated verbally or written in clinical notes and medical records.[20]

The Evolving Nature of Inclusive Language

As previously discussed, designations and preferences related to language change overtime. The fluid and ever-changing nature of inclusive language can lead to fear of speaking incorrectly or inappropriately. As a result, professionals may be hesitant to put forth ongoing effort to use inclusive language and may become defensive when faced with the knowledge that language once deemed appropriate may no longer be seen as acceptable. The complication of context in determining appropriateness introduces an additional layer of complexity as clinicians must not resort to simply substituting or swapping words but must also consider the nuances of the particular context in which the language is used.[3]

Strategies for Creating Environments that Support the Use of Inclusive Language

Ensuring that the entire dental team is participating in ongoing training related to inclusive language and communication is necessary. Self-reflection and self-awareness are the first steps in creating an inclusive environment for patients, for students, and for the entire dental team. Education and training should focus on *cultural humility*, an other-oriented concept characterized by "self-evaluation and critique, promotion of interpersonal sensitivity and openness, addressing power imbalances, and advancement of an appreciation of intracultural variation and individuality to avoid stereotyping."[32] Cultural humility differs conceptually from cultural competency in that cultural humility recognizes the fluid and heterogenous nature of culture and requires reflection on one's own beliefs and biases, as well as the impact these might have on interactions with patients. It has been argued that the language of cultural *competence* can connote the potential for mastery or achievement of a particular level of knowledge or skill.[33] Cultural *humility*, as a construct, places the "other" as the expert of their own cultural experience, considers intersectionality and centers the person within interactions and care. Cultural humility involves recognizing that one may be unsure about the language being used and being able to admit that one might not know or may be incorrect about terminology. A health care provider with cultural humility is willing to learn from patients about their experiences and is also aware of their own embeddedness within a particular culture(s).[33] Engaging in cultural humility promotes a growth mindset,[34] supporting the idea that we can all improve, which can mediate the fear, confusion, and defensiveness that clinicians and educators may feel when they are not sure what language to use or when they discover that social preferences have changed. Engaging in open discussions with colleagues and students about the use of inclusive language can encourage others to examine language with a critical eye and identify language and communication that could be improved to be more inclusive. Some studies have found that the use of gender-inclusive language, for example, is predicted by both deliberate and habitual processes.[35] Repeated and frequent use of inclusive language, as well as repeated and frequent practice in reflection on language, can habituate these skills so that they simply become part of what we do as clinicians and educators.

There are also procedural and organizational strategies that can be used to foster an environment where the use of inclusive language is prioritized. The use of scripts and standardized questionnaires for all clinical staff can help support development of skills related to use of inclusive language and can facilitate consistency in language use across the dental team.[36] Processes should be established for constant review of clinic materials, materials for patient education, and of curricular materials within dental education settings, with the aim of assessing and revising language used within these materials. Consulting with members of diverse communities to ensure that language is current and aligned with preferences and preferred community designations is advised. An even better approach is to bring in community members as integral members of review committees. Finally, and importantly, workplace and institutional policies that increase workplace diversity and representation of historically excluded or underrecognized groups within dentistry and dental education will create opportunities for inclusion of a broader number of voices and perspectives in these endeavors.

SUMMARY

Adopting inclusive language in dentistry is not just about adhering to politically correct terminology; it is a fundamental aspect of providing quality care that recognizes and respects the unique identities, experiences, and needs of all patients. Through person-first language and a commitment to understanding and respecting individual and community language preferences, dental professionals can create a more welcoming, empathetic, and effective health care environment. This approach fosters trust, enhances communication, and contributes to the overall goal of health equity by ensuring that every patient feels seen, heard, and valued. The challenge lies in overcoming structural biases and embracing the evolving nature of language, which requires ongoing education, reflection, and adaptation. By embedding inclusive language into all aspects of dental practice, from patient interactions to educational settings, the oral health care community can take significant strides toward a more inclusive and equitable health care system.

CLINICS CARE POINTS

- Use plain language to ensure clear, accessible communication for all patients.
- Actively listen to your patients to understand their preferred terms and language.
- Use person-first, non-stigmatizing language, placing the individual before their condition and using neutral descriptors.
- Maintain inclusive intake forms and documentation.
- Be open, continuously learn, and always approach patients with cultural humility in your communication.

DISCLOSURE

The authors have nothing to disclose.

REFERENCES

1. Marjadi B, Flavel J, Baker K, et al. Twelve tips for inclusive practice in healthcare settings. Int J Environ Res Publ Health 2023;20(5):4657.
2. Yuan S, Freeman R, Hill K, et al. Communication, trust and dental anxiety: a person-centred approach for dental attendance behaviours. Dent J (Basel) 2020;8(4):118.
3. Likis FE. Inclusive Language promotes equity: the power of words. J Midwifery Wom Health 2021;66(1):7–9.
4. NCCDPHP health equity glossary. CDC. Available at: https://www.cdc.gov/chronicdisease/healthequity/health-equity-communications/nccdphp-health-equity-glossary.html. Accessed February 27, 2024.
5. Calanan RM, Bonds ME, Bedrosian SR, et al. CDC's guiding principles to promote an equity-centered approach to public health communication. Prev Chronic Dis 2023;20:E57.
6. Johnson DD, Daum DN. Person-first Language in healthcare: the missing link in healthcare simulation training. Clinical Simulation in Nursing 2022;71:135–40.
7. Kwame A, Petrucka PM. A literature-based study of patient-centered care and communication in nurse-patient interactions: barriers, facilitators, and the way forward. BMC Nurs 2021;20:158.
8. Why Language Matters: Using Inclusive Language in the Workplace. Available at: Devry.edu. Accessed February 27, 2024 https://www.devry.edu/devryworks/thought-leadership/inclusive-language-in-the-workplace.html.
9. O'Daniel M, Rosenstein AH. Professional Communication and Team Collaboration. In: Patient safety and quality: an evidence-based handbook for nurses. Rockville (MD): Agency for Healthcare Research and Quality; 2008.
10. Zlatev J, Blomberg J. Language may indeed influence thought. Front Psychol 2015;6:1631.
11. Santiago PN, Konopasky AW, Railey KM. Words as windows: using Language to move toward an inclusive environment. J Grad Med Educ 2021;13(6):871–2.
12. Ruzycki SM, Holroyd-Leduc J, Chu P. The importance of developing and implementing an Inclusive Language and image policy in medical schools. Acad Med 2022;97(1):9.
13. Plain language materials and resources. CDC. Available at: https://www.cdc.gov/healthliteracy/developmaterials/plainlanguage.html. Accessed March 14, 2024.
14. Baires NA, Catrone R, May BK. On the importance of listening and intercultural communication for actions against racism. Behav Anal Pract 2021;15(4):1042–9.
15. Drwecki BB, Moore CF, Ward SE, et al. Reducing racial disparities in pain treatment: the role of empathy and perspective-taking. Pain 2011;152(5):1001–6.
16. Understanding Inclusive Language: A Framework. Berkeley CA: Berkeley Haas School of Business. Available at: https://haas.berkeley.edu/wp-content/uploads/Understanding-IL-Playbook-3.pdf. Accessed March 14, 2024.
17. Inclusive and gender-neutral language. NIH. Available at: https://www.nih.gov/nih-style-guide/inclusive-gender-neutral-language. Accessed March 14, 2024.
18. Botha M, Hanlon J, Williams GL. Does Language matter? Identity-first versus Person-First Language use in autism research: a response to vivanti. J Autism Dev Disord 2023;53(2):870–8.

19. Advancing Health Equity. A Guide to Language, Narratives, and Concepts. Washington, DC: AMA/AAMC; 2021.
20. Goddu A, O'Conor KJ, Lanzkron S, et al. Do words matter? Stigmatizing language and the transmission of bias in the medical record. J Gen Intern Med 2018;33(5): 685–91.
21. Merriam-Webster's Collegiate Dictionary. Available at: https://www.merriam-webster.com/. Accessed March 14, 2024.
22. Oxford English dictionary. Available at: https://www.oed.com/. Accessed March 14, 2024.
23. Flanagin A, Frey T, Christiansen SL, et al. The reporting of race and ethnicity in medical and science journals: comments invited. JAMA 2021;325(11):1049–52.
24. Rahman L. Disability Language guide. Palo Alto (CA): Stanford Disability Initiative Board; 2019.
25. Christiansen S, Iverson C, Flanagin A, et al. AMA Manual of Style: A Guide for Authors and Editors. 11th Edition. Chicago IL: Oxford University Press; 2020.
26. Herron CR. Inclusive Language matters: recommendations for health care providers to address Implicit bias and equitable health care. J Maine Med Center 2021;3(2):Article 9.
27. Lesbian, gay, bisexual, and transgender resource center. UCSF. Available at: https://lgbt.ucsf.edu/glossary-terms. Accessed March 14, 2024.
28. Nguemeni Tiako MJ, Ray V, South EC. Medical schools as racialized organizations: how race-neutral structures sustain racial inequality in medical education-a narrative review. J Gen Intern Med 2022;37(9):2259–66.
29. Berio L, Musholt K. How language shapes our minds: on the relationship between generics, stereotypes and social norms. Mind Lang 2023;38(4):944–61.
30. Mohamed SZ, Bourke L, Mitchell O, et al. 'It's a cultural thing': excuses used by health professionals on providing inclusive care. Health Sociol Rev 2022;31(1):1–15.
31. Zhao Y, Segalowitz N, Voloshyn A, et al. Language barriers to healthcare for linguistic minorities: the case of second language-specific health communication anxiety. Health Commun 2021;36(3):334–46.
32. Stubbe DE. Practicing cultural competence and cultural humility in the care of diverse patients. Focus (Am Psychiatr Publ) 2020;18(1):49–51.
33. Lekas HM, Pahl K, Fuller Lewis C. Rethinking cultural competence: shifting to cultural humility. Health Serv Insights 2020;13. 1178632920970580.
34. Dweck CS. Mindset: The New Psychology of Success. New York: Random House; 2006.
35. Sczesny S, Moser F, Wood W. Beyond sexist beliefs: how do people decide to use gender-inclusive language? Pers Soc Psychol Bull 2015;41(7):943–54.
36. Moore C, Dukes C. The value of identity: providing culturally-responsive care for LGBTQ+ patients through inclusive language and practices. Dela J Public Health 2019;5(3):6–8.

A Measure of Inclusion
Women as Authors in Oral Epidemiology and Dental Public Health, 2017-2022

Stefanie L. Russell, DDS, MPH, PhD[a],*,
Linda M. Kaste, DDS, MS, PhD, FAADOCR, FICD[b],
Shulamite S. Huang, PhD[c], Silvia Spivakovski, DDS[d]

KEYWORDS

• Gender • Equity • Inclusion • Women • Men • Diversity • United States • Dentistry

KEY POINTS

- While dentistry in North America has historically been dominated by men, gender representation in the profession is changing, with more than half of dental students being women since 2018.
- Dental Public Health is one dental specialty area that has rapidly and recently changed to comprise more women than men.
- Inclusion represents feeling welcome and participating in the environmental contexts of Diversity, Equity, and Inclusion.
- Other professions and disciplines regularly assess gender representation in publication authorship to measure gender equity and inclusion; however, fewer such assessments have been made in dentistry, especially in the United States.
- First and second authorship is predominantly held by women in the field of dental public health/oral epidemiology, however, senior authorship continues to be dominated by men, with little improvement in equity over time.

INTRODUCTION

In the United States and Canada, dentistry, such as medicine, has traditionally been male-dominated. In the United States, the proportion of women dentists has

[a] Department of Pediatric Dentistry and Community Dentistry, Rutgers School of Dental Medicine, 110 Bergen Street, Newark, NJ 07103, USA; [b] Department of Oral Biology, University of Illinois Chicago College of Dentistry, 801 South Paulina Street Room 569D MC 690, Chicago, IL 60612, USA; [c] Department of Epidemiology and Health Promotion, New York University College of Dentistry, 380 2nd Avenue, 3rd Floor Suite, New York, NY 10010, USA; [d] Department of Oral and Maxillofacial Pathology, Radiology and Medicine New York University College of Dentistry, 345 East 24th Street, Room 829, New York, NY 10010, USA
* Corresponding author.
E-mail address: stefanie.russell@rutgers.edu

Dent Clin N Am 69 (2025) 29–38
https://doi.org/10.1016/j.cden.2024.08.002
0011-8532/25/© 2024 Elsevier Inc. All rights are reserved, including those for text and data mining, AI training, and similar technologies.

increased to a point where currently they comprise 56% of first-year dental school students.[1] Some slow progress toward gender equity among dental faculty has been made, with an overall 16% increase seen in women as faculty members between 2011–2012 and 2018–2019, with women accounting for 37% of the full or part-time dental faculty workforce in 2018-19.[2] Clearly, gender gaps persist across dentistry, as seen both in academia[2–8] and in the general workforce.[9–11] Nonsurgical specialties of dentistry and those considered "primary care," including dental public health (DPH), tend to have a higher percentage of women than men entering the field.[4,12]

This article illustrates how measuring authorship by gender distribution can provide valuable data on inclusivity in dentistry. Considering inclusion as the feeling of being welcome in an environment, it provides the potential for an objective measurement of having access and being present, engaged, and involved. As such, we sought to measure gender in authorship in oral epidemiology and DPH publications over a six-year period and evaluate the impact of the COVID-19 pandemic on authorship gender equity.

Measuring Inclusion

One essential component of academic dentistry is "scholarly activity" as measured by research grant funding, presentations at international and national clinical and scientific meetings, and the quantity and quality of peer-reviewed publications. Indeed, publishing in scientific, clinical, or other academic journals is not only expected but necessary for academic advancement. Some investigators have measured gender equity in academic publishing and have identified gaps in disciplines with gender imbalance such as in medicine[13–15] and dentistry,[16–22] but also in areas with greater gender balance, including public health and its scientific foundation, epidemiology.[19,23]

As often seen in dentistry as well as general academia, women in dental academia face barriers that hinder their success, including unequal access to resources, gender bias, lack of women as role models, and sexual harassment that men in dental academia are unlikely or less likely to encounter.[4] An examination of whether women in dental academia are underrepresented might include a comparison of men to women proportions in various measures of academic success including academic position attainment, grant funding, and publishing.

To illustrate how one may measure inclusion or equity, we focus on gender equity. Gender, as compared with other constructs such as race, ethnicity, or sexual orientation, is a relatively straightforward construct to measure as gender is comparably easily identifiable through various methods. We focus on the dental specialty of dental public health (DPH) and its underlying science, oral epidemiology, as this specialty has a higher proportion of women compared to other specialties. We hypothesized that the higher proportion of women in the field of DPH would translate to gender equity in publications in journals that publish articles related to dental public health and oral epidemiology. We were also interested in whether an increasing trend over time for more women is seen for key (ie, first, second or senior) authorship positions, and whether factors including the gender of the journal editor-in-chief might be related to gender equity.

Data Source

We used PubMed to identify all journal articles published from January 2017 to December 2022 in the four primary English-language academic dental journals known to publish studies of oral epidemiology and DPH. These journals are *Community Dentistry and Oral Epidemiology*,[24] *Journal of Public Health Dentistry*,[25] *JDR Clinical and Translational Research*,[26] and *Community Dental Health*.[27]

Gender Measurement

We examined each article abstract (and/or the entire retrieved publication, if necessary), and manually extracted the first and last names of the first, second, and last (senior) author. Two investigators (SR and BS or SR and DS) independently identified the gender of each first, second, and last (senior) author (man vs woman vs unable to determine) using 3 methods: (1) as the DPH/oral epidemiology field is relatively small, and we often had first-hand knowledge of a person's gender because of personal or professional interactions or associations; (2) using academic, professional and other websites, and (3) by using the AI-online program "genderize" (*genderize.io*[28]), to identify gender based on the author first name. We then compared data on author gender between the two reviewers, and, in cases where there was discordance, we performed additional in-depth internet searches to reach a consensus. When no data were available on which we could make a definite judgment regarding the author's gender, we classified the gender as "unable to determine."

Analyses

Aside from author gender identification, for each publication, we assessed the following: (1) article title; (2) journal; (3) total number of authors; and (4) date of publication. We classified the type of each publication as either (1) original public health or oral epidemiologic research; (2) a systematic review of published epidemiologic or public health research; (3) another review of published epidemiologic or public health research; (4) editorial/opinion; (5) letter to the editor or author's response; (6) conference proceedings; (7) Erratum/Corrigendum; or (8) basic science/animal study/other (not epidemiologic or public health) research. We evaluated whether article type was related to women's authorship and subsequently excluded all articles other than original dental public health/oral epidemiology research articles from further analyses. We categorized the geographic location of the senior author as (1) North America; (2) Central/South America/Caribbean; (3) UK/Ireland; (4) Scandinavia/Nordic; (5) Europe; (6) Africa; (7) Middle East; (8) South Asia; (9) Southeast/East Asia; and (10) Australia/New Zealand.

We calculated the proportion of women as first, second, and last authors overall in the four journals more than the six years, and then by journal and year of publication using publication date (if the publication date was missing, we used the Epub date). We examined whether the proportion of women as first, second, and last authors changed over the six-years period and evaluated whether the articles published pre-vs. during/post-COVID-19 show differences. To do this, we excluded 2020 (since the COVID-19 pandemic officially began in March 2020) and defined 2017 to 2019 as the pre-pandemic era and 2021 to 2022 as the pandemic era. For bivariate analyses, we used chi-square tests, t-tests, and ANOVA. We used ANOVA to test trends over time. We used SPSS to conduct all statistical tests.

Evaluation

We identified 1483 publications from the four journals published between January 2017 and December 2022. The number of authors per publication ranged from 1 to 33 with a mean number of 4.87 authors (sd ± 2.70) and a median of 5 authors. We identified the gender of all but 0.7% (n = 11) of the first authors, 1.2% (n = 18) of the second, and 0.2% (n = 3) of the last authors. We treated these data as missing. We found that review articles were more likely to have women as authors for both the second and last author positions, relative to all original research articles and editorials ($P<.1$ for second authors and $P<.01$ for last authors) but found no statistically significant difference in the proportion of women authors in the first author position across article types. Follow **Fig. 1** to see which types of publications we excluded that led to the final dataset of 1147 original public health or oral epidemiologic research publications.

Proportion of women vs. men as authors
Overall, for the four selected journals over the six years period, we found that 59.6% of the first authors, 54.1% of the second authors, and 45.4% of the last authors were women. The proportion of women as authors by journal and year are presented in **Tables 1** and **2**.

Changes in percentages of women as authors over time
We identified increases over time in the proportion of women as authors in all author positions examined (first, second, and last). However, gains from 2017 to 2022 were more sizable among the second authors than the first and last authors (**Figs. 2 and 3**). The greatest increase in the proportion of women as authors from 2017 to 2022 came from the second author position, which increased by 6.5% points (signifying a 12.8% increase from 2017). In comparison, the proportion of women in the first author position increased from 2017 to 2022 by 3.6% points (6.0% increase from 2017), and in the last author position increased by 2.8% points (6.3% increase from 2017). However, only the changes across the years were statistically significant for the proportion of women as authors in the second author position.

We found sizable increases in the proportion of first and second women as authors in 2021 to 2022 (during the pandemic) relative to 2017 to 2019 (prepandemic). Pre-pandemic, the range of values for the proportion of women as first authors remained less than 60%. During the pandemic the range of values for the proportion of women as first authors was between 63% and 68%. Similarly, the proportion of women as second authors during the pre-pandemic period ranged between 51% and 52%, but during the pandemic, ranged between 57% and 58%. In contrast,

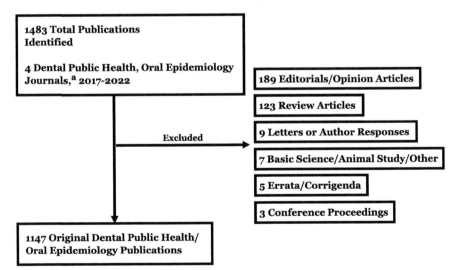

Fig. 1. Flow diagram, Article search results, Dental public health/oral epidemiology Journal Articles, 2017-2022. [a]Community Dentistry and Oral Epidemiology, Journal of Dental Public Health, Journal of Dental Research Clinical and Translational Research and Community Dental Health.

Table 1
Proportion of women as authors by journal, 2017-2022

Journal	Proportion of Women as Authors		
	First Author	Second Author	Last Author
Community Dentistry and Oral Epidemiology	60.4	53.5	44.4
Journal of Public Health Dentistry	61.0	56.6	45.9
JDR Clinical Translational Research	59.5	48.5	44.4
Community Dental Health	56.8	58.6	48.5
Total	59.6	54.1	45.4

the pre-pandemic period ranges for the proportion of women as senior authors overlapped with the during-pandemic ranges (44%–47% pre-pandemic vs 42%–47% during the pandemic).

Association of author gender with other factors
We evaluated whether there were differences in the proportion of women vs. men as first, second, and last authors by journal, by gender of the editor-in-chief at the time of publication, and by world geographic region. We found no statistically significant difference in the proportion of women as authors in the first or last author positions across journals with and without women as editors-in-chief. We did find statistically significant differences in the proportion of women as authors across world geographic positions across all authorship positions ($P<.01$ for all authorship positions examined). First authors were most likely to be women if they hailed from Africa (71.4%), Central/South America, and the Caribbean (68.6%) and North America (62.2%). First authors were least likely to be women if they hailed from Asia (49.2%) and Australia/New Zealand (51.5%). Last/senior authors were least likely to be women if they hailed from Africa (0%), Asia (28.6%), and the Middle East (33.3%).

DISCUSSION

We provide an example of how to measure gender inclusion in dental academia. We found an overall increase in gender equity over time in authorship in the DPH arena more than recently over the included six-years period an overall increase in gender equity over time over the included six-years period. Enthusiasm for this overall trend

Table 2
Proportion of women as authors by year for four journals, 2017-2022

Year	Proportion of Women as Authors		
	First Author	Second Author	Last Author
2017	59.6	50.6	44.4
2018	53.4	51.8	47.4
2019	57.8	51.3	43.9
2020	56.3	54.8	47.2
2021	67.9	58.7	42.1
2022	63.2	57.1	47.2
Total	59.6	54.1	45.4

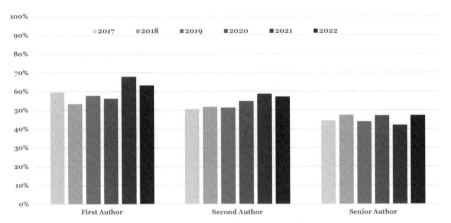

Fig. 2. Proportion of women as authors, dental public health/oral epidemiology, by year, 2017-2022.

toward gender parity, however, is tempered by our finding that changes have been slow and nonsignificant for the most important author positions (first and senior authorship). Given that we chose to evaluate a specialty of dentistry whereby women comprise a greater proportion of residents and faculty[29,30] than other areas of dentistry, particularly oral surgery,[31–33] these findings are alarming. We found that while women occupied the first and second authorship positions, men dominated and continued to dominate the senior author position as recently as 2022, the end of our study period.

This trend was also somewhat reflected when comparing the COVID-19 pandemic era to the pre-pandemic era, whereby we found no change in the senior author positions. The a trend toward an increase in women as first authors was dissimiliar to findings of other investigator who identified an increase in gender inequity during COVID-19 in the dental[34] and medical literature.[35,36] Our results contradict findings

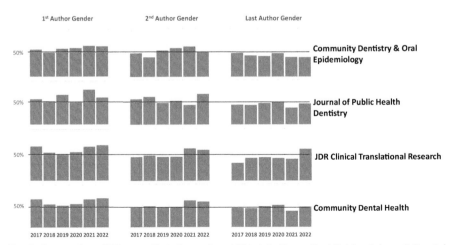

Fig. 3. Proportion of Women First, Second and Third Authors, Oral Epidemiology & Dental Public Health, by Year, 2017-2022.

that women's self-reported author and article submissions declined during the pandemic. Possible reasons include the long lag between submission and publication, that is, one may not see the full effects of the pandemic until we can gather years of data following the pandemic era.

We used several methods to measure the construct of gender. The DPH field is relatively small, and we relied on both our first-hand knowledge of a person's gender and/or internet searches of academic, professional, and other websites and/or the Artificial Intelligence (AI) online program "genderize" (*genderize.io*), to identify gender based on the author first name. In our case, the measurement of gender, compared with other constructs such as race or ethnicity, was relatively straightforward not only because we limited ourselves to two exclusive categories but also because we had three methods of identifying and/or confirming gender. Indeed, we had very little missing gender data and believe that our methods (use of multiple tools and independent evaluation by two investigators) resulted in negligible gender misclassification. One may use several web programs to measure gender, including "Gender API," NameAPI," "NamSor," and the Python package "gender-guesser," which can identify a person's gender given their first name, are valued for the determination of the gender of international names and are therefore especially useful for bibliographic analyses.[28] Several AI programs can also identify country of origin, ethnicity, and race.

Our evaluation has some limitations. First, author order is commonly listed according to the degree of involvement in the publication, with the last position used for the most senior person. While we assume that the last author is the supervisor, in some cases, the last author is merely an additional author who contributed to the article. However, if this were often the case, we would likely have seen more women listed as the last author, given the expectation that men continue to lead women in leadership roles in academia versus being last to be counted for contributions. In addition, in some cases, the first author is a person in the early stages of their career, for example, a student or resident. Given that over time, the DPH field has grown to have more women than men entering the field, seeing women as students in first and second authorship positions is not surprising.

Also, we did not measure several factors that might have been useful in explaining our results. For example, we did not attempt to measure the author's academic rank, which might have provided additional clues as to whether seniority was the reason for men's stronghold on senior authorship positions. Determining academic rank at the time of the article writing is a difficult task and would have required additional resources beyond the capacity of our research team at the time. Additional factors that should be included in future work include the gender of the Editor-in-Chief and the gender makeup of the editorial board and measures of work/life balance (which might have been particularly important during the pandemic), as well as such aspects as whether the author's partner is also a faculty member, stress levels, relationship dynamics, and number of children.

Inclusion may be defined as including and accommodating people historically excluded based on race, ethnicity, gender, sexuality, or ability. Evaluating gender in authorship positions provides an example of measuring inclusion. The Council of Science Editors promotes actions to "ensure DEI best practices and policies in scientific publishing" with "Collecting Demographic Data" as key metrics.[37]

SUMMARY

While we found that women comprise the majority of first and second authors, they lag behind men in senior authorship. This finding mirrors the conclusions of other investigations that have found that progress in reaching gender parity in leadership, particularly in academia, is slow. Given our findings, we echo others who have recognized the importance of mentoring and role models in providing opportunities for women to thrive not only as first and second authors but also in senior positions, as well as the importance of data for monitoring and evaluating the measurements of inclusion. Given our findings from both inside and outside the United States, the struggle for inclusion appears to be both a North American issue and a worldwide problem.

CLINICS CARE POINTS

- Measurement of inclusion and other aspects of DEI in dentistry has challenges, and the assessment of publication is one way of following trends.
- Representation of women as authors in DPH and Oral Epidemiology journals shows some progress in the inclusion of women in dentistry and scholarship activity.
- Ongoing actions are needed to ensure that the profession of dentistry is an inclusive environment for all its members.

DECLARATION OF AI AND AI-ASSISTED TECHNOLOGIES IN THE WRITING PROCESS

During the preparation of this work, the authors used "genderize.io" to identify gender based on the author's first name. After using this tool, the authors reviewed and edited the content as needed and took full responsibility for the publication's content.

ACKNOWLEDGMENTS

The authors acknowledge the efforts of Drs Belkys Saba (BS) and Diva Dhevamadhini Sundar (DS) who assisted in the gender identification of authors in the assessment.

DISCLOSURE

The authors have nothing to disclose.

REFERENCES

1. ADEA Trends in Dental Education, 2023–2024. Available at: https://www.adea.org/dentedtrends/. Accessed July 19, 2024.
2. Cain L, Brady M, Inglehart MR, et al. Faculty diversity, equity, and inclusion in academic dentistry: revisiting the past and analyzing the present to create the future. J Dent Educ 2022;86(9):1198–209.
3. Bompolaki D, Pokala SV, Koka S. Gender diversity and senior leadership in academic dentistry: female representation at the dean position in the United States. J Dent Educ 2022;86(4):401–5.
4. Garcia MN, Andrews EA, White CC, et al. Advancing women, parity, and gender equity. J Dent Educ 2022;86(9):1182–90.
5. Kim A, Karra N, Song C, et al. Gender trends in dentistry: dental faculty and academic leadership. J Dent Educ 2024;88(1):23–9.
6. Townsend JA, da Fonseca MA, Rodriguez TE, et al. Gender differences in pediatric dentistry chairs in the United States and Canada. J Clin Pediatr Dent 2020; 44(5):323–31.

7. Yuan JC, Lee DJ, Kongkiatkamon S, et al. Gender trends in dental leadership and academics: a twenty-two-year observation. J Dent Educ 2010;74(4):372–80.

8. Whelton H, Wardman MJ. The landscape for women leaders in dental education, research, and practice. J Dent Educ 2015;79(5S):S7–12.

9. Fleming E, Neville P, Muirhead VE. Are there more women in the dentist workforce? Using an intersectionality lens to explore the feminization of the dentist workforce in the UK and US. Community Dent Oral Epidemiol 2023;51(3):365–72.

10. Mertz EA, Bates T, Kottek A, et al. Practice patterns of postgraduate trained dentists in the United States. J Dent Educ 2022;86(9):1133–43.

11. Surdu S, Mertz E, Langelier M, et al. Dental workforce trends: a national study of gender diversity and practice patterns. Med Care Res Rev 2021;78(1_suppl):30S–9S.

12. Bates T, Jura M, Werts M, et al. Trends in postgraduate dental training in the United States. J Dent Educ 2022;86(9):1124–32.

13. Kim KY, Kearsley EL, Yang HY, et al. Sticky floor, broken ladder, and glass ceiling in academic obstetrics and gynecology in the United States and Canada. Cureus 2022;14(2):e22535.

14. Shah C, Tiwana MH, Chatterjee S, et al. Sticky floor and glass ceilings in academic medicine: analysis of race and gender. Cureus 2022;14(4):e24080.

15. Mueller C, Wright R, Girod S. The publication gender gap in US academic surgery. BMC Surg 2017;17(1):16.

16. Bernardi S, Fulgenzi MB, Rovera A, et al. Dentistry and gender gap: an overview of the Italian situation. Healthcare (Basel) 2023;11(6):828.

17. Consky EK, Bradshaw SM, Wein AN, et al. The proportion of female authors in oral and maxillofacial surgery literature has not changed in 20 years. J Oral Maxillofac Surg 2020;78(6):877–81.

18. Haag DG, Schuch HS, Nath S, et al. Gender inequities in dental research publications: findings from 20 years. Community Dent Oral Epidemiol 2023;51(5):1045–55.

19. Jones JE. Gender and research productivity in US and Canadian schools of dentistry. A preliminary investigation. Eur J Dent Educ 1998;2(1):42–5.

20. Reeves S, Loke WL, Mullerat-Pigem M, et al. 21st century gender trends of authorship in the British Journal of Oral and Maxillofacial Surgery. Br J Oral Maxillofac Surg 2022;60(7):978–82.

21. Sartori LRM, Henzel LT, de Queiroz ABL, et al. Gender inequalities in the dental science: an analysis of high impact publications. J Dent Educ 2021;85(8):1379–87.

22. Schumacher C, Eliades T, Koletsi D. Gender gap in authorship within published orthodontic research. An observational study on evidence and time-trends over a decade. Eur J Orthod 2021;43(5):534–43.

23. Chander S, Shelly S, Tiwana MH, et al. Racial and gender profile of public health faculty in the United States of America. Cureus 2022;14(5):e24998.

24. Community Dentistry and Oral Epidemiology. Available at: https://onlinelibrary.wiley.com/page/journal/16000528/homepage/productinformation.htm. Accessed July 19, 2024.

25. Journal of Public Health Dentistry. Available at: https://onlinelibrary.wiley.com/page/journal/17527325/homepage/productinformation.html. Accessed July 19, 2024.

26. JDR Clinical and Translational Research. Available at: https://journals.sagepub.com/home/jct. Accessed July 19, 2024.

27. Community Dental Health. Available at: https://www.cdhjournal.org/about-cdh. Accessed July 19, 2024.
28. Santamaría L, Mihaljević H. Comparison and benchmark of name-to-gender inference services. PeerJ Comput Sci 2018;4:e156.
29. Macek MD, Zavras A, Tomar SL, et al. American Board of Dental Public Health diplomate survey, 2021: competency domains and practice. J Publ Health Dent 2023;83(1):78–86.
30. Surdu S, Langelier M, Liu Y, et al. A national study of the practice characteristics of women in dentistry and potential impacts on access to care for underserved communities. Rensselaer, NY: Oral Health Workforce Research Center, Center for Health Workforce Studies, School of Public Health, SUNY Albany; 2019.
31. Bhalla N, Ravivarapu A, Dym H. Women in oral and maxillofacial surgery: population trends amongst residents. Oral Surg Oral Med Oral Path Oral Radiology 2022;134(3):e66.
32. Drew S. President's editorial women as oral and maxillofacial surgeons: past, present and future. Am Coll Oral Max Surg 2018. Available at: https://www.acoms.org/news/407850/Presidents-Editorial.htm. Accessed July 15, 2024.
33. Sayre K, Carver KZ, Anderson S, et al. Barriers to women in oral and maxillofacial surgery: a cross-sectional survey. J Oral Maxilofac Surg 2019;77(9S):e53.
34. Franco MC, Sartori L, Queiroz AB, et al. Impact of COVID-19 on the gender gap in dental publications: a retrospective cohort with three Brazilian journals. Braz Oral Res 2022;36:e0116.
35. Misra V, Safi F, Brewerton KA, et al. Gender disparity between authors in leading medical journals during the COVID-19 pandemic: a cross-sectional review. BMJ Open 2021;11(7):e051224.
36. Muric G, Lerman K, Ferrara E. Gender disparity in the authorship of biomedical research publications during the COVID-19 pandemic: retrospective observational study. J Med Internet Res 2021;23(4):e25379.
37. Council of Science Editors. 2.7 Diversity, Equity, and Inclusion in Scholarly Publishing. Available at: https://www.councilscienceeditors.org/2-7-diversity–equity–and-inclusion-in-scholarly-publishing. Accessed July 19, 2024.

Models of DEIB

Part I – Approaches to Inclusion from Other Health Professions for Consideration by Dentistry

Kendra M. Barrier, PhD, MSN, RN, CNE[a],
Demetrius J. Porche, DNS, PhD, APRN[a], Kendall M. Campbell, MD[b],
Tammi O. Byrd, RDH[c], Melanie Morris, LCSW[d],
Kate L. Blalack, MHR, MLIS[e], Candace Ziglor, DSW, LMSW[f],
Steph Tuazon, LCSW[g], Charles P. Mouton, MD, MS, MBA[h],
Janet H. Southerland, DDS, MPH, PhD[i],*

KEYWORDS

- Inclusion • Social work • Library science • Nursing • Medicine • Dental hygiene
- Dentistry • Interprofessional education

Continued

INTRODUCTION

Dentistry has evolved over time from a technical trade to a recognized health profession. The journey has been significant and marked by various changes in education, practice standards, research, and societal norms. This transformation has been impacted by technologic advances such as improved materials, advances in technology, digital imaging, and minimally invasive dental techniques. A better

[a] LSU Health Sciences Center New Orleans, School of Nursing, 1900 Gravier Street, New Orleans, LA 70112, USA; [b] Department of Family Medicine, University of Texas Medical Branch, 301 University Drive, Galveston, TX 77550, USA; [c] Portable Community Clinic, South Carolina, Columbia, SC, USA; [d] Department of Comprehensive Care, Tufts University, School of Dental Medicine, One Kneeland Street, Room 415, Boston, MA 02111, USA; [e] Digital Repositories, Library Applications Management, Hesburgh Libraries, University of Notre Dame, 271G Hesburgh Library, Notre Dame, IN 46556, USA; [f] University of Detroit Mercy, School of Dentistry, 2700 Martin Luther King Jr. Boulevard, Detroit, MI 48208, USA; [g] University of California, Los Angeles, Luskin School of Public Affairs Social Welfare, School of Dentistry – Special Patient Care, 337 Charles E Young Drive E, Los Angeles, CA 90095, USA; [h] Family Medicine, School of Medicine, University of Texas Medical Branch, 301 University Drive, Galveston, TX 77550, USA; [i] Oral and Maxillofacial Surgery, LSU Health Sciences Center New Orleans, 433 Bolivar Street, Suite 825, New Orleans 70112, USA
* Corresponding author. LSU Health Sciences Center, Suite 825, New Orleans, LA 70112.
E-mail address: jsouther@lsuhsc.edu

Dent Clin N Am 69 (2025) 39–53
https://doi.org/10.1016/j.cden.2024.08.007
0011-8532/25/© 2024 Elsevier Inc. All rights reserved, including those for text and data mining, AI training, and similar technologies.

Continued

KEY POINTS

- Dentistry has had marked changes in education, practice standards, research, and societal norms, with this transformation strongly impacted by technologic advances such as improved materials, advances in technology, digital imaging, and minimally invasive dental techniques.
- Dental education and the profession continue to be challenged with adequately addressing oral health disparities.
- Embracing inclusivity across the broader spectrum of dentistry and the health professions provides an opportunity to help create more parity and better oral health outcomes especially for marginalized populations.
- Diverse voices make for more enriching environments creating spaces for innovation, collaboration, and safety; perhaps other professions working with dentistry and leveraging evidence-based practices can assist with building more inclusivity across the dental profession.
- Dentists benefit from working with allied and other health professionals who each contribute their specialized knowledge and skills to effectively advance inclusion and belonging for and within the profession.

understanding of the relationship between oral and systemic health has helped to move the profession toward a more holistic approach to oral health care. Additionally, the expansion of interprofessional education (IPE) has broadened the scope of dentistry to encompass not just preventive oral health care but collaboration with other health care professionals to promote well-being and better overall health outcomes. While the incorporation of these areas into training and care delivery have been transformational for majority populations, dentistry as a profession has not been successful in closing substantial gaps in dental education, research, and care seen in more diverse and inclusive environments necessary to eliminate oral health disparities.

Poor oral health is often used as a measure of social inequity. The uneven distribution and challenges faced across the populations are closely aligned with lack of access and resources in underserved and rural communities. A variety of changes are needed to address the disparities that include resource allocation, social and public health policy, community organizations, access to dental care, and behaviors reflecting inclusion related to cooperation of individuals and dental professionals.[1] The history of dental education and the profession add challenges for addressing oral health disparities. Through embracing inclusivity across the broader spectrum of dentistry, an opportunity is created for more parity and better oral health outcomes especially for marginalized populations.[2] Dentistry is not without concerted effort focused on helping to shift this paradigm. Since the late 1970s, dental schools and dental professional organizations have developed and implemented programs aimed at creating the composition of students, faculty, researchers, and practitioners with the commitment to promote diversity, equity, inclusion and belonging (DEIB) within the profession.

The commitment to these efforts, however, has not been comparable across all programs and organizations, yielding less-than-optimal results. Furthermore, in 2024 a reversal in this trend of support has resulted in divestment of resources for diversity, equity, and inclusion (DEI) programming within certain states, especially their state-funded educational institutions and programs, which include dental schools. In the mist of this backward shift, it is imperative that a collective focus be held on the importance of health equity and social justice to oral health, which supports building of a dental workforce reflective of the communities served. Expanding efforts to embrace inclusivity across the dental profession requires collaborative efforts, not just within the profession but in conjunction with colleagues across the health professions.

This article explores approaches from other disciplines toward consideration of applications to creating inclusive and belonging environments in dentistry. The primary focus is on the opportunity for the dental professional to leverage content utilized by other health professions to enhance and expand inclusion efforts, and provide better experiences for learners, researchers, educators, and patients within dentistry. Examples are provided of activities, frameworks, and models that are portable and can serve to launch similar activities within dentistry. Selected models of inclusion covered in Part II of Models of DEIB from library science, medicine, nursing, dental hygiene, and social work can be used by the dental profession to help make more definitive strides toward inclusion to combat lack of access and inequitable oral health outcomes.

Interprofessional Education

IPE has become the standard in educating health professionals across disciplines to improve patient safety and better health outcomes.[3] Building highly effective health care teams is essential to delivering high-quality, safe, and patient-centered care.

Fostering collaboration, communication, and mutual respect among team members can optimize outcomes, enhance satisfaction, and promote a culture of excellence and continuous improvement in healthcare delivery.[4] The utilization of the tenets of IPE enhances inclusion through promoting collaboration, mutual respect, and understanding among healthcare professionals taking into consideration the many backgrounds and life experiences of practitioners and patients. IPE has also become a standard across curricula of health professional schools with competencies embedded across different disciplines.

The Interprofessional Education Collaborative (IPEC) emerged in 2009 as a result of the interest of six national education associations for health professions in advancing interprofessional learning across disciplines based on the premise that building high functioning health care teams was important to improve patient and population health outcomes. The professions initially participating included allopathic and osteopathic medicine, dentistry, nursing, pharmacy, and public health, now there are 21e affiliate health organizations. The panel, after forming, developed recommendations for competencies that help guide curriculum development to ensure proficiency required for this collaborative practice model (**Box 1**).[5] Version three of the competencies (released in

---

Box 1
IPEC core competencies 2009[5]

Values and Ethics Work with team members to maintain a climate of shared values, ethical conduct, and mutual respect.

Roles and Responsibilities–Use the knowledge of one's own role and team members' expertise to address individual and population health outcomes.

Communication–Communicate in a responsive, responsible, respectful, and compassionate manner with team members.

Teams and Teamwork–Apply values and principles of the science of teamwork to adapt one's own role in a variety of team settings.

2023) builds on the original work and framework recognizing variability across learners and institutions, refines competencies, and integrates concepts of the triple and quadruple aims.[6] The IPE model of training is a good example of how people from diverse backgrounds, different professions, levels of experiences, and interests can work together in a way that is meaningful and inclusive to realize better results.

LIBRARY SCIENCES
At Your Service

Cultural "competence" and cultural humility are parts of the health sciences disciplines with much of the research conducted within the medicine and education fields.[7] Librarians and archivists are a part of a larger ecosystem of public service, which parallels dentistry in the mission of service to community. One might attest that librarians play a part in the overall mental acuity and health of community members by providing resources for learning and educational growth: not only in intellectual pursuits and entertainment, but also entrepreneurship and wealth management, creative exploration and expression, and providing space for group gatherings, economic resources and public platforms.

When librarians think about "inclusion," it is difficult to separate it from their responsibility to be accountable and aware of the wide array of diversity needs across collective populations. Diversity includes, but is not limited to, age, ethnicity, neurobiologic variations, disabilities, and various levels of intellectual capabilities. However, *inclusion* is much more expansive in scope. Inclusion encompasses not only external community, but also internal community and the tools and resources are available. Inclusion means to be a part of, belong to, and actively contribute to an ecosystem's growth and evolution.[8–11] Inclusion also implies looking at not only diverse viewpoints and perspectives but also at how to apply these principles in a way that everyone feels welcome, provided for, and above all, *psychologically safe*. According to Davis and colleagues[12]:

> "A library that actually serves everyone takes care to think deeply and expansively about its spaces, services, and offerings and iterates with an expansive and diverse library user population in mind. I'm talking fat weight-rated chairs, fragrance-free policies, dimmed spaces for light sensitivity, multilingual staff with pay differentials for those skills, meaningful and accessible interpretation services, support for remote work, and more."[12]

Using this approach, the dental profession can more effortlessly address the challenges associated with accommodating the many different types of learners, providers, patients, and staff that make up the care team that can come from very different backgrounds and experiences.

The field of libraries lives and works in parallel universes. Information is not just about what is available in the microcosmic world of books and digital information; it is also about how the tacit world and knowledge are absorbed as if by osmosis. To create inclusive environments, it is important to understand biases that may serve as barriers to achieving inclusion and belonging. Schrodinger's Cat is used: to help look within the box to see how "set" practices might need to shift and evolve to include a larger view of reality.[13] The concept has been studied in the health care setting and has called into question the potential biases associated with decision-making in patient care associated with potential care outcomes.[13,14] One must be aware of what is known and what is not known, and what is yet to be known but is a possibility. This deeper introspection is needed as an aid to unravel the mysteries still underlying our commitment to achieving diversity and inclusion across health professions.

But what does it mean to *feel* included? Inclusion can be somewhat amorphous in reality. Everyone comes from intergenerational programming: having learnt certain behaviors from family, passed down so subtly that the effects are not known until adulthood. These experiences, both positive and negative, can cause implicit biases that create blind spots and gaps in understanding. Everyone has a certain idea of what reality entails, what *is* and what is *right* and *wrong*. Even though to believe eventual wisdom will be gained, this wisdom is based on experiences and what is noticed or even chosen to be paid attention to during those experiences. Diverse environments help dilute and color the bicameral, black and white thinking of the mind. Diverse voices add value by opening doors to those well-worn neuropathways, an example is provided in the following vignette in **Box 2**.

In this vein, equity can manifest in various forms: physical, structural, and in terms of information clarity. The primary categoric structures modeling the movement toward social maturity are diversity, equity, inclusion, and social justice, truncated as diversity, equity, inclusion and justice,[15,16] suggests the need for a model for transformation of organizational cultures to become fully functional in practice and ready to move into the future. Library sciences also incorporate Diversity Equity Inclusion and Accessibility (DEIA) recommendations and suggestions—bringing long-standing policies up to date.[17–19] Other ways that the library and archival fields have taken on the responsibility of being inclusive is to create international, national, and local strategic plans, vision statements, and initiatives that incorporate DEIA into the overall infrastructure and framework of the goals of the organization.

Key obligations and goals of any library organization is to provide information, with the *ethical* obligations of the American Library Association (ALA) being to ensure all voices are heard and *listened* to as expressed in the ALA ninth code of ethics (**Box 3**).[20]

Overall, the literature suggests that the movement must be a top tier effort supported by policy development and following a succinct strategic plan with *equity* as a focus. In practice, this must include outward movement into the community and a "cross pollination" of ideas, resources, and overall knowledge transfer.[15,16,21,22] The newest approaches move beyond the concept of "breaking down silos" into a rebuilding of community and a maturing of our overall organizational and environmental culture. In Darwinism, this approach is called "domestication." One genetic study did a fascinating experiment on pack behavior in dogs, learning that once an internal culture developed of "domesticity" or "calmness" newly introduced members had no choice but to conform to the new and evolved pack.[23]

Believing in the *good*—in the ability to adapt into kinder, more inclusive communities is on the rise, is learned that these methods work and, environments are created that

---

Box 2
Enhanced ways of seeing

Vignette
"There was a poster in the library where I used to work advertising a book and how important it was for development. It had a quote "my eyes could see no further...." and then the image of a book specifying that indeed they can when you choose to read. The very basis for the library is to enhance ways of seeing, to provide intellectual stimulation and growth, and perhaps escape for some of us, into a new world, to experience things we had not before." Feeling included means more than just feeling that the atmosphere of a building is calming and has suitable research space, or that the research collection we are viewing represents diverse voices, or even that our particular neurodiverse challenges have been assessed and accounted for in an online search engine."

Box 3
The ninth principle within the ALA code of ethics[20]

The ninth principle reads:

"We affirm the inherent dignity and rights of every person. We work to recognize and dismantle systemic and individual biases; to confront inequity and oppression; to enhance diversity and inclusion; and to advance racial and social justice in our libraries, communities, profession, and associations through awareness, advocacy, education, collaboration, services, and allocation of resources and spaces."

Specifics vary, for example, Northwestern Libraries Strategic plan includes the statement to: "Outfit library physical and digital spaces with visuals that mirror the demographics on campus through use of collections, exhibits or static imagery. Assess and prioritize the processing of collections that document diverse voices. Review descriptive language in online records for misleading, non-inclusive and offensive terminology on an ongoing basis. [and]

Identify funding sources to support the collection and processing of, as well as the outreach efforts related to, holdings that represent voices from historically marginalized groups."

---

people want to be a part of, with learning spaces that leave room for the "impossible" new thought or ways of experiencing and exploring history. Diverse voices provide a more enriching, beautiful tapestry of experiences. As a service profession librarians and archivists provide context, unaltered "truth" and a place for discovering whatever that means. Perhaps the start is not trying to identify a universal truth across all professions, but instead aiming at humility and identifying, however painful and shaming, historic and present accuracy.

MEDICINE
Points of Inclusion

The consideration of inclusiveness in medicine often focuses on situations or points of inclusion. Points of inclusion represent individual or person focused initiatives to ensure that people of all cultures and backgrounds are included in the organization. Inclusion follows diversity as diversity focuses on make-up of the people in the room, whereas inclusion focuses on engagement and contributions of people in the room, with a focus on interactions, team and collaboration. For purposes of the field of medicine, these people, or touchpoints of inclusion are defined in the broad categories of learners, faculty and staff, and senior leaders or administrators.

Learners

Learners are arguably the most important touchpoint for inclusion in academic health centers and in the field of medicine. Learners represent the future of care for a growingly diverse and aging population. Ensuring that diverse learners feel included in all aspects of their training, including having their cultures and backgrounds appreciated and their opinions heard and valued, is critical for learner growth and success. Learners in medicine can be defined as resident physicians, health professions students, graduate students, and medical students.

Opportunities to create inclusive environments are many for learners. Pathway programs are designed to do just that. These programs, often structured for marginalized or minoritized populations, can provide healthcare exposure and academic strengthening to the learner who were not afforded the opportunities or resources to maximize their learning and realize their potential because of systematic racism, community inequities, or socioeconomic concerns. Such programs, when structured appropriately with focused outcomes, can create inclusive environments and add diversity to the healthcare professional landscape.[24] Similar to these programs, holistic admissions processes in medical education bring inclusion and equity to a process that previously have advantaged some and disadvantaged others. Holistic admission allows for inclusion of groups who are important to the care of underrepresented and minority populations and can improve health outcomes.[25] Initiatives such as pathway programs and holistic admissions, while increasing the diversity of learners in medicine, are set up for creating inclusive environments for all learners to thrive and advance their education for the benefit of all patients.

Additional points of inclusion for learners include curricula that are developed from a culturally competent and culturally intelligent perspective.[26] These curricula consider the backgrounds and socioeconomic status of the learner and how those variables impact the learner's existence in the academic environment, and how equity is described in those environments to promote the success of all learners. These environments promote psychologic safety and inclusive excellence in a way that encourages the contributions and opinions of minoritized populations. In addition, mentorship programs focused on marginalized groups, and in particular cross-cultural mentoring programs, affinity groups, and support networks create an inclusive environment for learners promoting not only a diverse environment, but intersections in ways that can drive inclusive excellence.

Faculty and Staff

Inclusive excellence for faculty and staff members in medicine takes on a different approach than that of the learner. Faculty members tend to be long-term employees of the institution, with marginal turnover is marginal, maybe every four y or so. However, DEI efforts and efforts to promote an inclusive environment often receive limited attention. Importantly, academic environments must be inclusive, equitable, and nurturing to promote a collegial work culture that allows all to be successful and optimally productive. Part of creating this inclusion is through offices of faculty development. Increasing the skills of faculty and staff members who are marginalized or minoritized in medicine has the potential to increase their inclusion in the academic environment and their contributions across all missions of the institution. The setting of faculty development must be one of institutional equity in all areas of the academic environment, including areas such as education, clinical care, and research, along with identify focused development that considers impacts of culture and background. Other areas that impact inclusion are human resources (HR) and staff training. HR capture data on the makeup of the organization, to not only include training and degrees obtained, but also race/ethnicity and gender. By sharing the diversity makeup of the organization, HR gives a platform for inclusion for those who may be from marginalized or minoritized identities. Impacts of society-based initiatives or experiences such as minority physician focused organizations like the National Medical Association, the National Hispanic Medical Association, and the American Medical Women's Association not only provide pathways to increase diversity, but provide platforms for inclusion for minoritized physicians, impacting their roles in the healthcare environment, including those who work for academic health centers. Many of these organizations have institutions focused on affinity groups or support networks that support their inclusion and belonging.

Environments of Inclusion

Health systems
Academic health systems require an understanding of the health system environment and those who work to effectively create an inclusive culture. These academic health

systems are focused differently than the medical education environment, which centers primarily on the learner, curricula, and policies that govern and support education, the academic health system centers primarily on the patient, and require a broader and more structured approach to inclusion beyond but including learners, faculty, or staff. The focus on patients must appreciate how a patient's culture and background impact medical decision-making and approach-to-care. This requires the healthcare team to consider cultural beliefs and non-traditional medicines or treatments for certain conditions in conjunction with the patient to make unique and inclusive treatment plans as appropriate.

Community affiliates and community partnerships

The integration of the academic health system or medical school environment within the community in which it resides is an important engagement for both the community and health system. Historically, academic health systems' engagement consisted of gathering community data and creating community initiatives in the face of service;[27] in some instances, to only have them eventually dismantled, leaving the community let down bringing forth concerns of racism and lack of trust.[28,29]

Inclusion for community affiliates and community partnerships involves early and often engagement to build trust and relationships, such that academic health center leaders are present in the community and serve in ways to promote advancement of community goals. Community partnerships that are designed to be symbiotic with outcomes that evidence advancement on both fronts must exist. Excellence in inclusion includes dual representation on strategic planning, mission, and vision setting boards with key performance indicators and tangible outcomes that show a lasting impact on both the health system and the community.

NURSING
The American Association of Colleges of Nursing

The American Association of Colleges of Nursing (AACN) Diversity, Equity, and Inclusion Faculty Tool Kit defines inclusion as representing environmental and organizational cultures in which faculty, students, staff, and administrators with diverse characteristics thrive. Inclusive environments require intentionality and embrace differences, not merely tolerate them. Everyone works to ensure the perspectives and experiences of others are invited, welcomed, acknowledged, and respected in inclusive environments."[30] AACN[31,32] also defines belongingness as an effective state of engagement, one that heavily influences how people feel about themselves and others. Belongingness is a multifaceted and complex state of being that is heavily influenced by both internal and external factors. A students' sense of belongingness and their engagement in academic study have been identified as key contributors to student success.

When examining sense of belonging in the classroom setting, two major players emerge: faculty and classmates. Faculty set the tone for student interactions and model respect and valuing.[31–33] The extant literature shows that students with high levels of belonging speak to having had positive experiences with faculty who exhibit a caring disposition, use active learning techniques, and create safe spaces for expression and debate.[29] Institutional viability and capacity are necessary to examine the nursing school's infrastructure, allocation, and utilization of resources supporting alignment to build DEI capacity. Leadership, accountability, strategic planning, and metrics are key drivers of sustainability, excellence, transformation, and success. *Access and Success* provide nursing schools with opportunities to examine the structures, policies, practices, and attitudes to ensure access, retention, and success for all faculty, students, and staff. Access and success focus on access to nursing school, inclusion and belonging, and success of historically underrepresented and marginalized groups.

Fostering environments where diverse backgrounds are valued and respected is imperative for achieving mission-driven goals and commitments. Institutional *Culture and Climate* is critical to the experience of faculty, staff, and students, providing diverse, equitable, inclusive, and accessible environments where there is a collective sense of belonging and all individuals thrive and do their best work. *Education and Scholarship* are core competencies of nursing skills, reflecting faculty capacity, and pedagogical approaches that embody DEI. The structure of the processes determines the educational experiences of all students who are invited to participate in the learning environment.[33] **Fig. 1** provides a visual depiction of the Inclusive Excellence Ecosystem for Academic Nursing.[31]

National League for Nursing

In 2006, the National League for Nursing (NLN) defined diversity as "affirming the uniqueness of and differences among persons, ideas, values, and ethnicities". The integration of diversity and inclusion was considered an essential element to achieve a state of inclusive excellence in which diverse faculty, staff, and students are able to flourish. This culture of inclusive excellence is expected to encompass behaviors across academic and health care systems.[34] The inclusion of a representative nursing workforce that resembles the patient population has been demonstrated to improve patient and overall health care outcomes. NLN called for nursing educational programs to develop this culture of inclusion.

The NLN framework addresses two broad areas–administrative leadership, as well as faculty and staff leadership is expected to emphasize the academic mission,

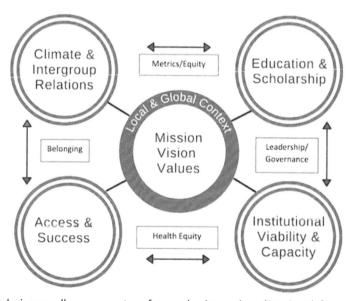

Fig. 1. Inclusive excellence ecosystem for academic nursing. (Reprinted from Toward a Model of Inclusive Excellence and Change in Post-Secondary Institutions. by Williams. D.A., Berger, J.B., & McClendon, S. A. Published by the American Association of Colleges and Universities, 2005, https://inclusionandbelongingtaskforce.harvard.edu/publications/toward-model-inclusive-excellence-and-change-postsecondary-institutions.)

leadership, students, staff, and curricular matters. Institutions need to move beyond simply the creation of mission statements that address diversity to the development of a campus culture and climate that embodies and embraces inclusive excellence. The development of a diversity plan is considered a strategy to achieve the level of integration required for institutional level culture and climate of inclusive excellence. The institution's administrative leadership team should resemble the student population. This should be achieved by recruiting a diverse administrative leadership team. A strategy to promote the development of a diverse leadership team is the creation and implementation of minority focused leadership institutes or programs.[34,35]

A diverse nursing faculty and staff workforce further promote an environment of inclusion and belonging within the academic environment. Parallel to the need for a representative leadership team, faculty, and student body, a representative student body that resembles the health care population is needed. Just as patients relate to health care providers that resemble them, students likewise feel a sense of belonging with the presence of faculty and staff that look like them. To achieve diversification of the nursing workforce, comprehensive plans to focus on the recruitment and retention of diverse student populations should exist. These plans should assure that students are not only admitted but retained to the point of academic program completion and transition into practice. A diverse student body brings into the academic institution a population of students with various life experiences, backgrounds, and learning styles. The development and implementation of inclusive student-centered pedagogies are essential to the promotion of student engagement.[34,36,37]

DENTAL HYGIENE

Comprehensive preventive care is important to addressing oral health disparities and involves engaging the entire oral health care team. Dental hygienist professionals have the potential to greatly improve outcomes and save populations from pain and suffering. They are the primary members of the dental team charged with patient education and disease prevention in the dental office. They can also, if utilized at the top of their training, be instrumental in removing barriers to care by delivery of preventive services outside the office within the community.

Individual and community level socioeconomic factors (insurance type and community-level education attainment) and receipt of dental procedures explain a large share of the observed racial and ethnic disparity in the risk of tooth decay among racially and ethnically minoritized children and adolescents.[38] Dental hygienists delivering comprehensive preventive care in variety of community settings are cost-effective and will broaden access to care for marginalized populations and improve oral health care outcomes. This approach also has the potential to increase inclusivity across educational and practice settings.

Dental Hygiene Practice

The profession of dental hygiene graduated the first class of professionals November 17, 1913, due to a demand for "these women in public institutions such as schools, hospitals, and sanitoriums."[39] Times have changed, and dental practices have evolved into group practices and large corporate practices, but the majority are still independent solo private settings. The role of the dental hygienist has also changed since inception to be more of a "prevention specialist." This model of practice varies depending on the state, but the primary model requires the dental hygienist to be supervised by the dentist. Newer laws passed across the country have expanded the scope of practice allowing for greater and even independent practice. While these enhancements in dental hygiene practice have better addressed challenges with access to dental care and prevention in underserved and rural areas, there remains some tension between the national organizations of dentistry and dental hygiene that have caused some conflicting opinions related to the level of independence that should be afforded to a hygienist. With such discord, there is still a need for a dental practice model that embraces diversity at all levels, and that is extended to team members, as well as patients is a step in the right direction.

Dental Public Health Hygienists and Accessibility

Access to preventive dental services is critically important to improving health literacy within patient populations and communities to help improve oral health outcomes. Allowing hygienists to be able to work at the top of their education and licensure would provide broader patient access; however, this strategy is still a source of great controversy and debate among the dental team. Dental hygienists along with advocating for greater autonomy have also included work in public health settings as needed for prevention and to reduce disease burden. While the dental team functions as a unit in practice, the dentist/dental hygiene dynamic does not always result in inclusion. The vignette illustrates an example of how professional dynamics can limit creating inclusive environments within dentistry with resolution sometimes from outside of dentistry (**Box 4**).

SOCIAL WORK

Healthcare has changed in recent years. No longer is the expertise of a single provider enough to provide the best care; instead, there has been a movement toward collaborative, co-located, and integrated service models.[40] Dentistry has been slower in embracing integrated care and continues to take steps to improve in this area. One way dentistry has embraced integrated care is by including social workers on their teams, specifically in dental schools.

Box 4
Challenges of inclusion in dental hygiene practice

Vignette
   In 2003, a State Board of Dentistry (BOD) was charged with restraining the trade of dental hygiene and depriving children of care for the actions it took against Health Promotion Specialists (HPS–Dental Hygienist), a portable community program that was serving schools in the state. These charges resulted in a guilty verdict against the BOD by the United States Department of Justice and 10 years of sanctions against the Board in 2007. The Federal Trade Commission (FTC) commented that "there was a conflict of interest when a regulatory board is dominated by individuals that have a vested economic interest in controlling the licensure, education, and practice of another profession it regulates." The FTC also stated that "there is no evidence that allowing dental hygienists to provide preventive services without supervision is a safety issue." The FTC further argued that "restricting the practice, without evidence that the restriction limits public safety, unnecessarily reduces competition." As a result of the investigation and findings, in January 2018, the BOD approved dental hygienists providing comprehensive preventive services in the state. Grant funding, training and equipment was provided to 41 registered dental hygienists and the faculty of the dental hygiene programs in August 2018.

United States. Federal Trade Commission. Statutes and decisions pertaining to the Federal Trade Commission. Washington :United States Government Printing Office. FTC Matter/File-Number 0210128; Docket Number 9311.

The first social worker introduced into dentistry was in the late 1940s at the University of Chicago to conduct psychosocial assessments of a family's readiness for dental care.[41] In 1960, a dentist and dental educator proposed establishment of Departments of Social Dentistry in dental schools.[42] This department would be responsible for developing curriculum, teaching, and research on the social and behavioral aspects of delivering patient care. In 1983, a social worker with dual appointments in both social work and dental schools developed a conceptual model of social work in dentistry. This model expanded previous ideas of social dentistry by directly naming the need for social workers to be in this role and including a direct service component of assessment, interventions, case management, advocacy, and interdisciplinary collaboration.[43] Since then, social work and dental colleagues have collaborated to establish social work's role as part of interprofessional teams in oral health settings by highlighting the biopsychosocial spiritual aspects of oral health and addressing the impact of social and structural determinants on understanding, accessing, and utilizing care.[44–49]

While the discussion of the need and value of social workers in dental education is not new, today only 20 out of 73 (27.4%)[46] accredited dental schools in the United States were identified to have active social work departments or services. Social workers are uniquely positioned to be effective members of integrated dental teams. Barriers to dental care, such as material hardships, lack of transportation, and intersecting social complexities, are intervention points for social workers. By leveraging their expertise in psychosocial risk factors, conducting behavioral health assessments and interventions, prioritizing culturally sensitive service adaptation, and applying theoretic frameworks through a social justice lens, social workers can promote oral health equity and contribute to delivering high-quality, patient-centered care.[47]

SUMMARY

Dentistry traditionally is a profession that provides comprehensive oral health care across the life span. Inclusion is important in dentistry to effectively leverage all team members to optimize the care of patients, educate future providers, and create innovative approaches to oral health care for all members within the population. The dental profession must be inclusive to form collaborations with other health professionals in recognition of the impact of oral health on overall health and the need for medical dental integration to care for those with uncomplicated dental care, as well as those with complex medical and dental needs. See of the article "Models of DEIB: Part II–Exploring Models of Inclusion from other Health Professions for Dentistry", where selected models and frameworks successfully used in other health professions that potentially could serve as an accelerant to help dentistry create more opportunities for promoting inclusion and belonging within the profession ranks are described.

CLINICS CARE POINTS

- A variety of existing models and frameworks developed and implemented by national health professional organizations, as well as others are available for use in education, research, and patient-care settings that focus on inclusion.
- Dentists should explore more opportunities through "open access", as well as other venues to leverage the specialized knowledge and skills of colleagues, for it is incumbent on dentists

to understand the scope and practice of other professions to better serve patients from all backgrounds.

- The models suggest approaches by other health professions that can go a long way in potential transformations of dental education and practice with ultimately improving oral health outcomes especially for marginalized and vulnerable populations.

- As oral health inequities continue to impact communities disproportionately, a need exists for reimbursement models of dental care focused on a collaborative approach centered on care coordination, quality-of-care, and health equity.

DISCLOSURE

The authors have nothing to disclose. There were no funding obtained or conflicts to disclose.

REFERENCES

1. Northridge ME, Kumar A, Kaur R. Disparities in access to oral health care. Annu Rev Publ Health 2020;41:513–35.
2. Mills A, Berlin-Broner Y, Levin L. Improving patient well-being as a broader perspective in dentistry. Int Dent J 2023;73(6):785–92.
3. Bosch B, Mansell H. Interprofessional collaboration in health care: lessons to be learned from competitive sports. Can Pharm J (Ott) 2015;148(4):176–9.
4. O'Leary N, Salmon N, Clifford AM. 'It benefits patient care': the value of practice-based IPE in healthcare curriculums. BMC Med Educ 2020;20:424.
5. Interprofessional Education Collaborative. Core competencies for interprofessional collaborative practice: 2016 update. Washington, DC: Interprofessional; 2016. Education Collaborative. Available at: Core Competencies for Interprofessional Collaborative Practice: 2016 Update. (Accessed 29 May 2024).
6. Interprofessional Education Collaborative. IPEC core competencies for interprofessional collaborative practice: version 3. Washington, DC: Interprofessional Education Collaborative; 2023. Available at: IPEC Core Competencies for Interprofessional Collaborative Practice: Version 3 (memberclicks.net). Accessed May 29, 2024.
7. Goodman XY, Nugent RL. Teaching cultural competence and cultural humility in dental medicine. Med Ref Serv Q 2020;39(4):309–22.
8. Knology Research Organization, What neurodivergent patrons want from small and rural libraries, Available at: https://programminglibrarian.org/articles/what-neurodivergent-patrons-want-small-and-rural-libraries, (Accessed 29 May 2024).
9. Vacek R., Jaffer N., Adler R., From siloed to connected: using engagement as a means to improve the culture of a library division, 2022; Available at: https://dx.doi.org/10.7302/4383. (Accessed 29 May 2024).
10. Kulikauskionė K. The concept of socially inclusive library in changing society. Socialiniai tyrimai 2019;42(1):67–78.
11. Kulikauskiene K, Liukinevičienė L. The theoretical model of an inclusive library for people with disabilities and its practical implementation. Izzivi prihodnosti 2020; 5. https://doi.org/10.37886/ip.2020.005.
12. Davis N, Vaden M, Seiferle-Valencia M, et al. The library is NOT for everyone (yet): disability, accommodations, and working in libraries. College Research Libraries News, [S.l.] 2024;85(2):58. Available at: https://crln.acrl.org/index.php/crlnews/article/view/26204/34145. Accessed May 29, 2024.

13. Schrödinger Erwin. Die gegenwärtige Situation in der Quantenmechanik (The Present Situation in Quantum Mechanics). Naturwissenschaften 1935;23(48): 807–12.

14. d Alencar Neto JN, Farina E, Nunes Sampaio MC. Schrödinger's Cat bias: a new cognitive bias proposed. Cureus 2021;13(1):e12697.

15. Sadvari J, Quill T, Scott D. Practicing map and geospatial information librarianship through the lens of diversity, equity and inclusion, and justice. J Map Geogr Libr 2022;18(1–2):143–7.

16. Leung SY, McKnight L, editors. Knowledge justice. Cambridge, MA: The MIT Press; 2021.

17. Kang Q, Lu J, Wang P, et al. A systematic review of IDEAs in librarianship: working together move toward greater ideas. J Librarian Inf Sci 2024. https://doi.org/10.1177/09610006241230104.

18. Northwestern Libraries. Diversity, equity, inclusion and accessibility at the libraries. Available at: https://www.library.northwestern.edu/about/administration/deia-at-the-libraries.html. Accessed May 1, 2024.

19. Northwestern University Libraries. Strategic plan — diversity, equity, inclusion and accessibility at the libraries. Available at: https://www.library.northwestern.edu/documents/about/nul_deia_strategicplan2021_external_final.pdf. Accessed April 1, 2024.

20. American Library Association. Available at: https://www.ala.org/news/member-news/2021/07/ala-adopts-new-code-ethics-principle-racial-and-social-justice. Accessed April 1, 2024.

21. Geiger L, Mastley CP, Thomas M, et al. Academic libraries and DEI initiatives: a quantitative study of employee satisfaction. J Acad Librarian 2023;49(1):1–10.

22. Pun R, Kubo H. What collaboration means to us: advancing equity, diversity, and inclusion initiatives in the library profession. Collaborative Librarianship 2022;13(1): Article 2. Available at: https://digitalcommons.du.edu/collaborativelibrarianship/vol13/iss1/2. Accessed July 12, 2024.

23. Wilkins AS. A striking example of developmental bias in an evolutionary process: the "domestication syndrome". Evol Dev 2020;22:143–53.

24. Taylor S, Iacobelli F, Luedke T, et al. Improving health care career pipeline programs for underrepresented students: program design that makes a difference. Prog Community Health Partnersh 2019;13(5):113–22.

25. Snyder JE, Upton RD, Hassett TC, et al. Black representation in the primary care physician workforce and its association with population life expectancy and mortality rates in the US. JAMA Netw Open 2023;6(4):e236687.

26. Sternberg RJ, Siriner I, Oh J, et al. Cultural intelligence: what is it and how can it effectively Be measured? J Intell 2022;10(3):54.

27. Wilkins CH, Alberti PM. Shifting academic health centers from a culture of community service to community engagement and integration. Acad Med 2019;94(6): 763–7.

28. Togioka BM, Duvivier D, Young E. Diversity and discrimination in health care. Treasure Island, FL: StatPearls Publishing; 2024. Available at: https://www.ncbi.nlm.nih.gov/books/NBK568721/. Accessed July 12, 2024.

29. Hamed S, Bradby H, Ahlberg BM, et al. Racism in healthcare: a scoping review. BMC Publ Health 2022;22(1):988.

30. AACN diversity, equity & inclusion faculty tool Kit. The American Association of Colleges of Nursing. AACN Diversity, Equity, and Inclusion (DEI) Tool Kit, designed in 2021, for nursing faculty to guide schools on DEI efforts. Available at: https://www.aacnnursing.org/diversity-tool-kit. Accessed May 29, 2024.

31. Carter BM, Sumpter DF, Thruston W. Overcoming marginalization by creating a sense of belonging. Creativ Nurs 2023;29(4):320–7.
32. Gayle BM, Cortez D, Preiss RW. Safe spaces, difficult dialogues, and critical thinking. Int J Scholarsh Teach Learn 2013;7(2):Article 5.
33. Williams DA, Berger JB, McClendon SA. Toward a model of inclusive excellence and change in post-secondary institutions. Washington DC: Association of American Colleges and Universities; 2005. Available at: Toward a Model of Inclusive Excellence and Change in Postsecondary Institutions (du.edu). (Accessed 29 May 2024).
34. National League of Nursing. Achieving diversity and meaningful inclusion in nursing education: a living document from the national League for nursing. 2016. Available at: https://www.nln.org/docs/default-source/uploadedfiles/professional-development-programs/vision-statement-achieving-diversity.pdf. (Accessed 29 May 2024).
35. Relf MV. Advancing diversity in academic nursing. J Prof Nurs 2016;32(55):S42–7.
36. Ahn R, Ingham S, Mendez T. Socially constructed learning activity: communal note-taking as a generative tool to promote active student engagement. Transformative Dialogues 2016;8(3):1–15.
37. Ahn R, Class M. Student-centered pedagogy: Co-construction of knowledge through student-generated midterm exams. IJTLHE 2011;23(2):269–81.
38. Choi SE, White J, Mertz E, et al. Analysis of race and ethnicity, socioeconomic factors, and tooth decay among US children. JAMA Netw Open 2023;6(6):e2318425.
39. Fones AC. Read before the section on mouth hygiene, preventive dentistry and public health at the 7th international dental congress Philadelphia, PA. August 24, 1926. American Dental Hygienists' Association 2013;87(suppl 1):58–62.
40. Heath B., Wise Romero P. and Reynolds K., A standard framework for levels of integrated healthcare. SAMHSA-HRSA Center for Integrated Health Solutions, 2013. Available at: https://thepcc.org/sites/default/files/resources/SAMHSA-HRSA%202013%20Framework%20for%20Levels%20of%20Integrated%20Healthcare.pdf (Accessed 1 May 2024).
41. Wexler P, McKinley E. Function of a social worker in Walter G. Zoller Memorial Dental Clinic, University of Chicago Clinics. J Dent Educ 1953;17(2):59–66.
42. Blackerby P. Why not a department of social dentistry. J Dent Educ 1960;24:197–200.
43. Rao AP. Social work in dentistry. Health Soc Work 1983;8(3):219–29.
44. Doris JM, Davis E, Du Pont C, et al. Social work in dentistry: the CARES model for improving patient retention and access to care. Dent Clin North Am 2009;53(3):549–59.
45. Zerden LS, Morris M, Burgess-Flowers J. Oral health and social work integration: advancing social workers' roles in dental education. Health Soc Work 2023;48(1):43–53.
46. Findley PA, Weiner RC. Oral health across the life course: a role for social work. J Stud Soc Sci Humanit 2020;6(1):10.
47. Kirkbride JB, Anglin DM, Colman I, et al. The social determinants of mental health and disorder: evidence, prevention and recommendations. World Psychiatr 2024;23(1):58–90.
48. Flick K, Marchini L. The interprofessional role in dental caries management. Dent Clin North Am 2019;63(4):663–8.
49. Petrosky M, Colaruotolo LA, Billings RJ, et al. The integration of social work into a postgraduate dental training program: a fifteen-year perspective. J Dent Educ 2009;73(6):656–64.

Models of Diversity, Equity, Inclusion, and Belonging

Part II—Exploring Models of Inclusion from Other Health Professions for Dentistry

Kendra M. Barrier, PhD, MSN, RN, CNE[a],
Demetrius J. Porche, DNS, PhD, APRN[b], Kendall M. Campbell, MD[c],
Tammi O. Byrd, RDH[d], Melanie Morris, LCSW[e],
Kate L. Blalack, MHR, MLIS, CA, DAS[f], Candace Ziglor, DSW, LMSW[g],
Steph Tuazon, LCSW[h], Charles P. Mouton, MD, MS, MBA[i],
Janet H. Southerland, DDS, MPH, PhD[j],*

KEYWORDS

- Models • Social work • Library science • Nursing • Medicine • Dental hygiene
- Dentistry • Inclusion

KEY POINTS

- Existing models and frameworks of inclusion have been developed and are available for use in education, research, and patient care settings.
- Models of inclusion from other health professions can be considered for adaptation and implementation in dentistry to promote more inclusive environments.
- Dentists should explore more opportunities through "open access" as well as other venues to leverage the specialized knowledge and skills of colleagues.

Continued

[a] LSU Health Sciences Center New Orleans, School of Nursing, 1900 Gravier Street, New Orleans, LA 70112, USA; [b] LSU Health Sciences Center New Orleans (LSU Health – New Orleans), School of Nursing, 1900 Gravier Street, New Orleans, LA 70112, USA; [c] Department of Family Medicine, University of Texas Medical Branch, 301 University Drive, Galveston, TX 77550, USA; [d] Portable Community Clinic, South Carolina, 125 Laurel Branch Way, Columbia, SC 29212, USA; [e] Department of Comprehensive Care, Tufts University, School of Dental Medicine, One Kneeland Street, Room 415, Boston, MA 02111, USA; [f] Library Applications Management, Hesburgh Libraries, University of Notre Dame, 271G Hesburgh Library, Notre Dame, IN 46556, USA; [g] University of Detroit Mercy, School of Dentistry, 2700 Martin Luther King Jr. Boulevard, Detroit, MI 48208, USA; [h] University of California, Los Angeles, Luskin School of Public Affairs-Social Welfare, School of Dentistry Special Patient Care, 337 Charles E Young Drive East, Los Angeles, CA 90095, USA; [i] Family Medicine, School of Medicine, University of Texas Medical Branch, 301 University Drive, Galveston, TX 77550, USA; [j] Oral and Maxillofacial Surgery, LSU Health Sciences Center New Orleans, 433 Bolivar Street, Suite 825, New Orleans, LA 70112, USA
* Corresponding author. Louisiana State University, 433 Bolivar Street, Suite 825, New Orleans, LA 70112.
E-mail address: jsouther@lsuhsc.edu

Dent Clin N Am 69 (2025) 55–68
https://doi.org/10.1016/j.cden.2024.08.010   dental.theclinics.com

Continued

- The models suggested while not all encompassing can provide pathways for continued transformation of the culture of dental education to ultimately improve oral health outcomes especially for marginalized and vulnerable populations.
- As oral health inequities continue to impact marginalized communities disproportionately, reimbursement models are needed for collaborative approaches centered on care coordination, quality of care, and health equity.

INTRODUCTION

Dentistry as a profession has over the last decade continued to expand efforts to promote diversity and inclusion. With significant changes in the makeup of learners and aging of the population, including practitioners, it has become clear that in order to be more competitive and patient centered, dentistry must better incorporate and embrace the concepts of diversity and inclusion to effectively educate and care for future generations. The American Dental Association along with other national dental organizations has outlined their approach to diversity and inclusion through their respective committees, strategic plans, and toolkits.[1–3]

The focus of this article is to explore potential models and frameworks from other professions that can be adopted across academic institutions, professional organizations, communities, and practices to further enhance inclusion and belonging in dentistry. The opportunity to transport models and frameworks developed by other professionals, who have been more active in this area, can potentially expedite the movement toward social justice and health equity for dentistry and oral health while incorporating broader perspectives to influence change and transformation.

MODELS FROM OTHER HEALTH PROFESSIONS
Library Sciences

Open information

The *"Open Access"* to information is one way to level the playing field and create inclusivity to provide access in a broader way than has been done before. Around the world, people are waking up to the idea that for researchers, scientists, *or really anyone*, to be accountable for their actions, information must be open and accessible. The silos of the world are coming down in the hope that we might one day be "global citizens". Some countries in the world are opening up information accessibility creating avenues for inclusion and belonging. In 2022, the White House Office of Science and Technology Policy issued a memorandum that all federally funded research would need to become "open access" by December 2025.[4] This edict, known as the *Nelson Memo*, created an uproar in the world of science and information. Perhaps this, more than any other initiative, created space to show inclusivity, braveness, and belief that to have progress many eyes, opinions; and ways of thinking must be involved. In addition, several innovative models have been created within the library science arena from conferences convened in 2021 and 2023, crafting a multifaceted way to advance diversity and inclusion. These models are highlighted by an international platform for open access and a manual helping to dispel diversity as two dimensional and binary. The overarching agreement from the discussions is that inclusiveness provides a way of creatively putting oneself in the place of another.[5,6]

Toolkits and guides

On a more library-specific level, the library and archival professions have been working hard on developing effective strategies for combating non-inclusive and exclusive access to information and environments. Countless libraries have instituted cultural competence training and specialized focus groups to implement practices and help create both formal and informal ways of making sensitivity to others part of organizational culture. In other cases, they provide specific strategies for implementing practices, via toolkits or checklists. Vacek, Jaffer, and Adler[7] provide practices such as workshops, implementing trans-appropriate design, and social groups for discussion in a non-formal way.

Similarly, libraries are creating online toolkits on inclusive collection development to help identify hidden voices in existing collections and/or voices and literature that has been omitted from the collections due to bias, aiding in more diversified and inclusive information sources. Often these also include ways to implement these practices in both digital and physical spaces.[8]

MEDICINE

When considering models of inclusion the goal in medicine, as in any profession, is to move toward inclusive excellence. Inclusive excellence is a journey in ensuring that diversity, equity, and inclusion are incorporated in all aspects of the academic environment and that equity exists for all.[9] It is recognizing that the success of the organization depends on the diversity and inclusion of its members and that engaging, valuing, and encouraging all members, including those with marginalized or minoritized identities, are a must for the optimization of the organization. Two models are shared along with our own designed figure that demonstrates structural needs to promote diversity, equity, inclusion, and belonging (DEI) in academic environments. Also, the need for preparatory work that provides underpinning and breaks down barriers to success is incorporated. Barriers that need overcoming include the minority tax, gate blocking of faculty, institutional racism, and the impacts of historical injustices against minoritized people no matter the profession.[10–12]

Addressing these barriers makes it clear that there are foundations that are critical for any model of inclusion. Building on this foundation also requires an understanding of needed actions to move organization toward inclusion, after creating a diverse environment, but before attempts at inclusive excellence.[13] Steps are defined toward creating an inclusive environment. **Fig. 1** demonstrates a pathway from diversity to inclusion in a way that is measurable and delineates outcomes that build toward inclusive excellence.

Marjadi and colleagues[14] provide a model of inclusion for inclusive practice in the health care setting from medicine that includes multiple domains of inclusion involving

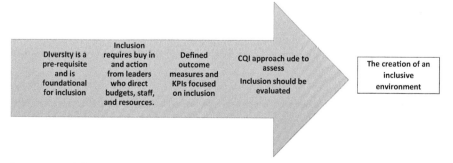

Fig. 1. Toward the creation of an inclusive environment: a model from medicine.

advocacy, education, commitments, signage, language, inclusive built environments, and inclusive labeling. The model presents five underpinning concepts with inclusion as the center in which they define tips that promote inclusion in the health care environment (**Fig. 2**). Another model of inclusion from medicine takes on a departmental approach within the academic health center and provides a model for others to follow if seeking to create a committee to focus on diversity, equity, and inclusion. Lingras and colleagues[15] provide six considerations for creating a departmental-based DEI committee, which they formed in a department of psychiatry.

The first part of this departmental approach is ensuring support from institutional leadership, followed by a process that leads to guideline creation and ongoing evaluation. The belief is that such models as shown in **Fig. 3**,[15] bring forward critical elements of inclusion. They not only include the programming and acts of making sure that diversity is included in the academic environment, but commonalities speak to the need for committed leadership and ongoing evaluation as important to ensuring a true inclusion that is evidenced by an equitable work environment as described by those who are marginalized or minoritized in the organization.

NURSING

A diverse nursing faculty and staff workforce promote an environment of inclusion and belonging within the academic environment. Parallel to the need for representative

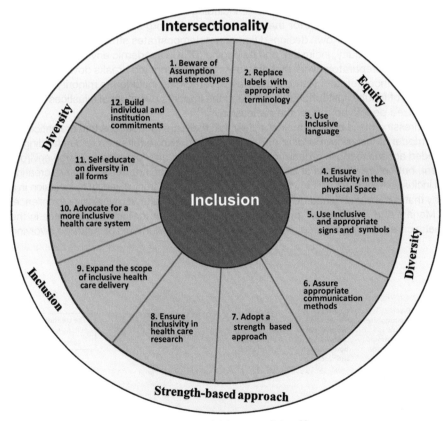

Fig. 2. Adapted model of inclusion: a model from medicine.[14]

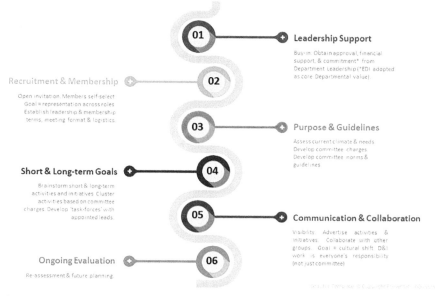

A Model for Developing a Departmental Diversity, Equity, & Inclusion (DEI) Committee

01 — **Leadership Support**
Buy-in: Obtain approval, financial support, & commitment* from Department Leadership (*EDI adopted as core Departmental value).

Recruitment & Membership — **02**
Open invitation. Members self-select. Goal = representation across roles. Establish leadership & membership terms, meeting format & logistics.

03 — **Purpose & Guidelines**
Assess current climate & needs. Develop committee charges. Develop committee norms & guidelines.

Short & Long-term Goals — **04**
Brainstorm short & long-term activities and initiatives. Cluster activities based on committee charges. Develop 'task-forces' with appointed leads.

05 — **Communication & Collaboration**
Visibility: Advertise activities & initiatives. Collaborate with other groups. Goal = cultural shift. D&I work is everyone's responsibility (not just committee).

Ongoing Evaluation — **06**
Re-assessment & future planning.

Fig. 3. Developing departmental based DEI: a model from medicine.[15]

leadership teams and faculty, a representative student body that resembles the health care population is needed as well. Just as patients relate better to health care providers who resemble them, students likewise feel a sense of belonging in the presence of faculty and staff.

To achieve diversification of the nursing workforce, comprehensive plans to focus on the recruitment and retention of diverse student populations are needed. These plans should assure that students are not only admitted but retained to the point of academic program completion and transition into practice. A diverse student body brings into the academic institution a population of students with various life experiences, backgrounds, and learning styles. The development and implementation of inclusive student-centered pedagogies are essential to the promotion of student engagement (**Box 1**) and expanding capacity in the workforce.[16] The inclusive excellence framework developed by the National League of Nursing outlines components

---

Box 1
Student-centered pedagogies that promote inclusion: a model from nursing[16]

Student-centered pedagogies
- Multisensory approaches that include visual, auditory, kinesthetic, and tactile
- Active participation structures
- Communal note-taking
- Student learning communities
- Long-term memory strategies such as mnemonics
- Breaking content down to promote absorption overtime—chunking
- Formative informal assessments
- Metacognition strategies such as reflection

essential for recruiting and retaining a diverse student body and workforce. Implementation of the framework by academic leaders in dentistry along with faculty and staff could provide a more comprehensive approach to promoting inclusive environments within the dental profession (**Fig. 4**).[17–20]

The American Organization for Nursing Leadership (AONL) also has developed guiding principles that are consistent with their organizational mission, the American Nurses Association Code of Ethics for Nursing, and the Future of Nursing 2020 to 2030 recommendations. **Fig. 5** presents the AONL DEIB principles and strategies/action steps.[20] Additionally, AONL has been able to influence leadership practice and development through the establishment of leadership competencies. Leadership competencies are the knowledge, skills, and abilities expected for effective leadership.[20] These leadership competencies are expected of nursing leaders in various roles such as nurse executive, chief nurse executive, post-acute care, nurse manager, and nurse executive in population health. The opportunity for application of these competences in dentistry to potentially assist academic and organizational leaders is compelling as the challenges of building inclusive spaces within the dental profession continue.

These leadership competencies consist of six leadership domains—communication and relationship building, leadership, knowledge of the health care environment and clinical principles, professionalism, business skills and principles, and the leader within. Three of the six leadership competency domains have sub-domains of knowledge, skills, and behaviors expected for diversity, equity, inclusion, and belonging.[16]

Stages of Psychological Safety: Defining the Path to Inclusion and Innovation

Having psychological safety is a key element in developing inclusive spaces allowing effective communication and collaboration. Movement through successive stages of

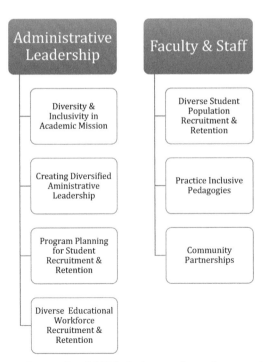

Fig. 4. National league for nursing (NLN) inclusive excellence framework.[19]

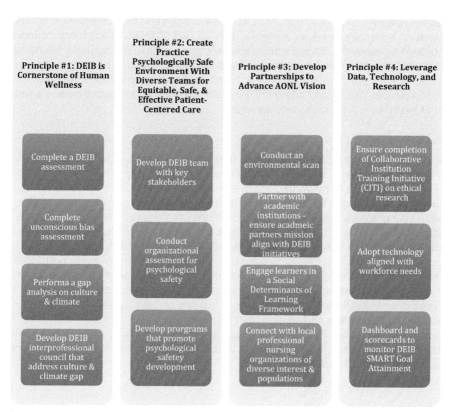

Fig. 5. American Organization for Nurse Leadership diversity, equity, inclusion, and belonging (DEIB) principles and strategies.[19]

psychological safety includes the following stages: Stage (1) inclusion safety; Stage (2) learner safety; Stage (3) contributor safety; Stage (4) challenger safety; there is also consideration of another stage that would involve avoiding paternalism and exploitation.[21] The first stage is member safety, where the team accepts the members and grants them shared identity. Identified next is learner safety, the second stage, which indicates the member feels safe to ask questions, experiment, and even make mistakes. Next is the third stage of contributor safety, where the member feels comfortable participating as an active and fully vested member of the team occurs. Finally, the fourth stage of challenger safety allows the member to take on the status quo without repercussion. The benefits that can be gleaned from having safe spaces are associated with wellness, for individuals and organizations, authentic expression in display of self, and higher performance. Access to social scientists as organizational consultants for dental professionals can provide a firsthand framework to help build and establish psychological safety, creating environments where individuals feel included, fully engaged, and encouraged to contribute their best efforts and ideas.

DENTAL HYGIENE

Oral health can increase inclusivity across medical, dental, and community settings when dental hygienists are allowed to work to the top of their education and licensure.

Dental hygienists can work clinically as well as to involve and train other health professionals on minimally invasive care techniques as part of an interdisciplinary inclusive approach to caring for diverse populations and their needs. The focus of the dental profession should continue exploring and understanding how building an inclusive culture across the oral care team and other health professions can reduce the burden of dental diseases-associated morbidity using comprehensive preventive care in a variety of health care and community settings.

Minimally Invasive Care

Minimally invasive oral health care seeks to preserve and remove as little of the tooth as possible. This dental strategy seeks to preserve the integrity of tooth structure and prevent oral disease from progressing to more severe stages. Such conservative care is an approach that can be performed by the dental hygienists as well as other trained health care professionals in clinical and community settings broadening opportunities for access to oral health care for those overburdened with oral disease. The outlined examples of minimally invasive care in **Box 2** provide proven strategies that can be applied by the dental hygiene professional to be more productive but also better integrated into the education and practice of dentistry. The expertise of the dental hygienist can be leveraged for training others in and outside health care to help expand access to oral health care in countless ways, building on team and inclusive practices. Extending opportunities and sharing techniques among health care members to learn about, with, and from each other as well as other professions provide a notable example for modeling interprofessional education (IPE) and collaborative practice leading to improved care outcomes.

Box 2
Materials and techniques for team, collaborative practice, and access: a model from dental hygiene

Atraumatic restorative technique (ART)
- "ART" is a maximally preventive and minimally invasive approach to manage and arrest further progression of a carious lesion.
- Selective caries removal with hand instruments or without carious lesion removal may be implemented depending on the case, before placing materials to seal the carious lesion and arrest the disease progression to restore form and function to a tooth.
- Use of glass ionomer is a bonus in that the material recharges its fluoride content when a patient uses a fluoride toothpaste.
- ART is painless and without anesthetic or drilling.

Intermediate restorative technique (IRT)
- This technique's basics are the same as ART
- However, becomes IRT when a provider needs the patient to return or be referred for final restoration of a tooth with different materials.

Silver diamine fluoride
- The material is a clear liquid that combines antibacterial effects of silver and the remineralizing effects of fluoride as a therapeutic agent for managing and preventing cavities.
- Arrest active carious lesions painlessly.

Silver modified restorative technique
- The basic techniques are the same as ART
- However, prior to placement of the glass ionomer, silver diamine fluoride is placed over the cavity/carious lesion.

SOCIAL WORK
Integrated Social Work in Dental Education Model

Since 2019, the Social Work in Dentistry (SWID) network has existed, when it was established by social workers in dental education to provide peer support and advance the role of social work in the dental field. Part of advancing the role of social work has been discussing the implementation of social work services or training at each dental institution. Members of SWID represent 20 different dental schools across the nation in diverse geographic areas. Although each dental school integrates social work based on their specific student and patient needs, some of the communal areas of integrating social work in dental education would further enhance inclusivity wholistically across the profession.

Direct Clinical Practice in Dentistry

One of the main roles of social work in dental education is providing direct clinical services to the dental patient. Either through patient or dental provider referral, social workers are called into the clinic setting to provide interventions focused on mitigating a range of social needs that are barriers to dental care, such as dental anxiety, substance use, transportation needs, and psychoeducation on the dental treatment. Social workers can also assist with dental-related care coordination. For example, a patient not connected to a primary care provider (PCP), but needs a medical clearance to continue with dental care, not having a PCP in this case could be a barrier to completing treatment.

This practice borrows from medical social work in addressing the holistic needs of patients. Social workers utilize a biopsychosocial model that improves both patient care and interdisciplinary support by enhancing dental teams' sensitivity and responsiveness to their patients' complex life circumstances.[18,22] Social workers also use a person-centered care model in dentistry, focusing on comprehensive care strategies that address dental needs and the accompanying social and health issues.[23] Such models are particularly effective in managing acute and chronic health and social complexities, improving the quality of care and patient satisfaction, ultimately contributing to better health outcomes and reduced inequities.

Dental Education and Social Work—Didactic Education

Dental schools have embedded social workers in faculty or staff roles to fulfill curriculum requirements in didactic education. Each dental school is unique in the population that it services and its subsequent needs. As such, the didactic content social workers provide is unique across schools. The content all fits under the umbrella of person-centered care[24] or the ability to provide individualized care to a person using the biopsychosocial spiritual model.[25] This model posits that people are complex and can only be understood if we look at all the factors that make up a person biologically, psychologically, socially, and spiritually.[26] This requires a dental student to stop focusing solely on the mouth and instead take a step back and look at the patient as an entire person. Social workers train dental students to reflect on how their positionality impacts how they provide care, as well as how their patients' lived experiences may impact their ability to understand and address their health.[22] This includes training related to cross-cultural communication, bias, and microaggressions to help dental students see their patients through a different lens.

Social workers also provide education in the public health model of dentistry and understanding how social determinants of health might impact a patient and, subsequently, their treatment or access to treatment.[23] One in 5 people experience a mental illness, so dentists will likely work with someone who has a diagnosable mental illness.[24] Social workers teach dental students and residents to understand the signs and symptoms of these mental illnesses, how to connect a person with resources for assistance, and potential modifications to make when working with this patient.[26]

Communication skills are paramount in being an excellent dental practitioner and achieving person-centered care.[27,28] Social workers educate dental students and residents on how to hone communication skills to provide excellent chairside manner, using active and reflective listening skills, empathy, compassion, and radical acceptance to better understand patients and their needs[28]; when trainees know their patients' needs, they can better meet them. Dental students can do this through skills such as motivational interviewing to assess their patients' motivation to address their health needs.[29,30]

Social Work Education—Practicum Supervisor

Social workers in dental education may be social work student practicum supervisors. As a practicum supervisor, they conduct weekly supervision meetings, administer daily tasks, and provide professional development opportunities. For example, social work students, both bachelor's and master's level, are trained to assess and discuss the social needs of dental patients and identify appropriate resources to meet these needs. Part of the way that social work students assist dental students is by exploring their patient's holistic needs and providing resources or other support for the patients. This support can increase patients' likelihood of disclosing areas of need or concern, and models to dental students how they can work collaboratively with other health professions and address needs themselves.[30,31]

Community Engagement

In identifying barriers to care, social workers aim to reduce oral health disparities by enhancing access to dental care through community engagement and partnerships. Since social workers interface with many community agencies and providers either as a referral source, resource, or care partner for patients, they have been able to identify new opportunities to collaborate with the community to enhance oral health and present new opportunities to the dental school.[32] For example, social workers may be able to identify a local community that may benefit from oral health education, such as information events on best hygiene practices or when to go to the dentist versus the emergency room. Social workers can coordinate events focused on dental students and faculty providing oral health screenings and evaluations for community members seeking dental care.

Recommendations for the Continued Inclusion of Social Work in Dentistry

Although considerable progress has been made in integrating social work into dental education, ongoing efforts are required to sustain and deepen this integration. SWID represents a collaboration across systems capable of making impacts at the individual, community, and larger system levels. Accordingly, social workers advocate for recommendations tailored to each of these levels to further advance the integration of social work within dental practice and education. Similar to their counterparts in health care, dentists benefit from aligning with other professionals who each contribute their specialized knowledge and skills to advance patient care. Dentists need to be comfortable working interprofessionally. To leverage the specialized knowledge and skills of social workers, it is incumbent on dentists to understand the scope and practice of SWID to understand their value to an oral health team for both the patients they serve and the professionals they work with. This teamwork of interprofessional collaboration works best when professionals understand each other's roles and show mutual respect.[33]

Social workers can significantly improve patient care experiences, helping dentists meet their patients' varied needs. Effectively collaborating with social workers requires taking the steps to engage at the level of patient care. While working in this manner is second nature for newer social workers, these graduates have been exposed to nontraditional spaces and gained collaborative skills during their education, while those who are more senior may need to expand understanding to intentionally help shift the paradigm to become valued members of the oral health care team. Once these steps are taken, we collectively can begin to develop more standardized care practices together with dental colleagues that address social determinants of health and disease and help promote health parity and inclusivity.

Since oral health inequities continue to impact marginalized communities disproportionately, reimbursement models are needed for dental care focused on a collaborative patient-centered approach for care coordination, quality of care, and health equity involving other providers.[34] The field of dentistry can advocate for an accountable care organization model for dentists, in which social work services would be part of the financing system and where, rather than fee-for-service, payment is based on care quality performance.[35] Exploration of refining this model is still needed empirical to build literature on the social work integration in oral health care.

SUMMARY

Like their counterparts in the health professions, dentists benefit from working with allied and other health professionals who each contribute their specialized knowledge and skills to effectively advance inclusion and belonging within the profession. Various models and frameworks have been developed and implemented by national health professional organizations, academic institutions, libraries, and departments available for use in dental settings of education, research, and patient care. Dentists should explore more opportunities through "open access" as well as other venues to leverage the specialized knowledge and skills of colleagues; it is incumbent on dentists to understand the scope and practice of other professions to better contribute to promoting environments of inclusion and belonging.

While improvements in the dental curriculum are already benefiting new graduates embracing concepts of inclusion, those graduates who are not exposed to these concepts may need to look for training programs to help them better understand and apply principles of inclusive practices within their respective areas of influence. The models suggested while not all encompassing can potentially go a long way in transforming the culture of dental education and improving oral health outcomes especially for marginalized and vulnerable populations.

CLINICS CARE POINTS

- Involving other professions representing diverse educational backgrounds and health care workforce members can help promote an environment of inclusion and belonging within institutions and communities to improve oral health inequities.

- These models suggested can be useful in improving the culture of dental education and oral health outcomes especially for marginalized and vulnerable populations.

- Dentists benefit from working with allied and other health professionals who each contribute their specialized knowledge and skills to effectively advance inclusion and belonging across the professions.

- The models and frameworks displayed represent national professional organizations, academic institutions, libraries, and departments work that are available for use as exemplars for dentistry in education, research, and patient care settings to promote more inclusive spaces.

DISCLOSURE

The authors have nothing to disclose.

REFERENCES

1. American Dental Association. Advancing Inclusion while Growing Membership Diversity 2020-2025. Diversity and Inclusion Strategy. Available at: https://www.ada.org/-/media/project/ada-organization/ada/ada-org/files/about/ada_diversity_inclusion_plan.pdf. (Accessed 29 May 2024).
2. Schwartz SB, Smith SG, Johnson KR. ADEA faculty diversity toolkit: a comprehensive approach to improving diversity and inclusion in dental education. , J Dent Educ 2020;84(3):279–82.
3. International Association for Dental Research. Diversity, Equity, Inclusion, Accessibility, and Belonging Statement. 2023. Available at: Diversity, Equity, Inclusion, Accessibility, and Belonging Statement | IADR - International Association of Dental Research. (Accessed 1 July 2024).
4. Yale Library Guides. Open access: library statement on the Nelson Memo. Available at: https://guides.library.yale.edu/c.php?g=296385&p=9596444. Accessed May 1, 2024.
5. International Association of Libraries and Institutions. IFLA ARL section's "Inclusiveness through openness" conference proceedings. 2023. Available at: https://www.ifla.org/news/ifla-arl-sections-inclusiveness-through-openness-conference-proceedings-now-available/. Accessed April 15, 2024.
6. International Council of Archives, Section on archives and human rights. Available at: https://www.ica.org/ica-network/professional-sections/sahr/sahr-newsletters/. Accessed April 29, 2024.
7. Vacek R, Jaffer N, Adler R. From siloed to connected: using engagement as a means to improve the culture of a library division. Available at: https://deepblue.lib.umich.edu/handle/2027.42/172234. Accessed April 29, 2024.
8. Berkeley Library Guides, Diversity, equity and inclusion in earth & planetary science: follow diverse voices, Available at: https://guides.lib.berkeley.edu/geo_dei/voices (Accessed 22 April 2024), 2024.
9. Murray TA, Benz MR, Cole B, et al. The journey toward inclusive excellence. J Nurs Educ 2023;62(4):225–32.
10. Geier TJ, Timmer-Murillo SC, Brandolino AM, et al. History of racial discrimination by police contributes to worse physical and emotional quality of life in black americans after traumatic injury. J Racial Ethn Health Disparities 2024;11(3):1774–82.
11. Nuriddin A, Mooney G, White AIR. Reckoning with histories of medical racism and violence in the USA. Lancet 2020;396(10256):949–51.
12. Amaechi O, Foster KE, Tumin D, et al. Addressing the gate blocking of minority faculty. J Natl Med Assoc 2021;113(5):517–21.
13. Mullin AE, Coe IR, Gooden EA, et al. Inclusion, diversity, equity, and accessibility: from organizational responsibility to leadership competency. Healthc Manage Forum 2021;34(6):311–5.

14. Marjadi B, Flavel J, Baker K, et al. Twelve tips for inclusive practice in healthcare settings. Int J Environ Res Publ Health 2023;20(5):4657.

15. Lingras KA, Alexander ME, Vrieze DM. Diversity, equity, and inclusion efforts at a departmental level: building a committee as a vehicle for advancing progress. J Clin Psychol Med Settings 2023;30(2):356–79.

16. Ahn R, Class M. Student-centered pedagogy: Co-construction of knowledge through student-generated midterm exams. IIJTLHE 2011;23(2):269–81.

17. Hughes R, Meadows M, Begley R. AONL nurse leader competencies: core competencies for nurse leadership. Nurse Leader 2022;20(5):437–43.

18. Gayle BM, Cortez D, Preiss RW. Safe spaces, difficult dialogues, and critical thinking. Int J Scholarsh Teach Learn 2013;7(2).

19. American Organization of Nurse Leaders (AONL). AONL Guiding principles: diversity, equity, inclusion and belonging toolkit. 2024. Available at: https://www.aonl.org/system/files/media/file/2024/02/AONL_Diversity-Toolkit_2024.pdf. Accessed May 29, 2024.

20. National League of Nursing. Achieving Diversity and Meaningful Inclusion in Nursing Education: A Living Document from the National League for Nursing 2016. Available at: https://www.nln.org/docs/default-source/uploadedfiles/about/vision-statement-achieving-diversity.pdf?sfvrsn=85a4d30d_0. (Accessed 29 May 2024).

21. Clark TR. The 4 stages of psychological safety: defining the path to inclusion and innovation. Berrett-Koehler Publishers; 2020. Available at: https://web-p-ebscohost-com.lsuhscno.idm.oclc.org/ehost/detail/detail?vid=0&sid=024b5578-3b32-4d47-bb6b-19785ebf81f2%40redis&bdata=#AN=2254408&db=e000xna. Accessed April 28, 2024.

22. Davis N, Vaden M, Seiferle-Valencia M, et al. The library is not for everyone (Yet): disability, accommodations, and working in libraries. Coll Res Libr News 2024;85(2):58. ISSN 2150-6698. Available at: https://crln.acrl.org/index.php/crlnews/article/view/26204/34145. Accessed July 12, 2024.

23. Ao H, Deng X, She Y, et al. A biopsychosocial-cultural model for understanding oral-health-related quality of life among adolescent orthodontic patients. Health Qual Life Outcome 2020;18(1):86.

24. Lee H, Chalmers NI, Brow A, et al. Person-centered care model in dentistry. BMC Oral Health 2018;18(1):198.

25. Scrambler S, Delgado M, Asimakopoulou K. Defining patient-centred care in dentistry? A systematic review of the dental literature. Br Dent J 2016;221(8):477–84.

26. Vermette D, Doolittle B. What educators can learn from the biopsychosocial-spiritual model of patient care: time for holistic medical education. J Gen Intern Med 2022;37(8):2062–6.

27. Petrosky M, Colaruotolo LA, Billings RJ, et al. The integration of social work into a postgraduate dental training program: a fifteen year perspective. J Dent Educ 2009;73(6):656–64.

28. Moore R. Maximizing student clinical communication skills in dental education—a narrative review. Dent J 2022;10(4):57.

29. Morris M, Atterbury E, Minichetti C, et al. Patient-dental student provider communication in an academic dental clinic setting: a dyadic data analysis. J Dent Educ 2023;87(11):1585–93.

30. Gillam DG, Yusuf H. Brief motivational interviewing in dental practice. Dent J 2019;7(2):51.

31. Oral Health in America: Advances and Challenges [Internet]. Bethesda (MD): national institute of dental and craniofacial research(US); 2021 Dec. Section 4, oral health workforce, education, practice and integration. Available at: https://www.ncbi.nlm.nih.gov/books/NBK578298/. Accessed April 28, 2024.
32. Lee H, Chalmers NI, Brow A, et al. Person-centered care model in dentistry. BMC Oral Health 2018;18(1):198.
33. Ansa BE, Zechariah S, Gates AM, et al. Attitudes and behavior towards interprofessional collaboration among healthcare professionals in a large academic medical center. Healthcare (Basel) 2020;8(3):323.
34. Northridge ME, Kumar A, Kaur R. Disparities in access to oral health care. Annu Rev Publ Health 2020;41:513–35.
35. Mayberry ME. Accountable care organizations and oral health accountability. Am J Publ Health 2017;107(S1):S61–4.

Advancing Dentistry Through Respectful Inclusion: A Focus on Racial Inequities

Eleanor Fleming, PhD, DDS, MPH, FICD[a],*,
Herminio L. Perez, DMD, MBA, EdD[b]

KEYWORDS

- Inclusion • Workforce • Students • Faculty • Climate • Health equity • Dentistry
- Racism

KEY POINTS

- Diversifying dentistry is key to realizing oral health equity.
- Support of inclusive climates at dental schools and within professional dental organizations is crucial to the recruitment and retention of diverse people.
- Inclusive communication and the use of person-centered language should be leveraged for advancing population-level health and promoting optimal clinical outcomes in working with patients and communities.
- Sentiments such as "I don't see color" do not support inclusive environments and result in the "othering" of people, which fails to create belonging.
- Dentistry requires building inclusive leadership capacity to support belonging and diversity.

INTRODUCTION

Dentistry faces challenges in expanding its ranks to include diverse people (specifically, minoritized people).[1,2] For groups like American Indian/Alaska Native, Black, Hispanic, Native Hawaiian and Pacific Islanders, their presence in dentistry has not grown significantly over the decades.[3,4] Although dental schools have an accreditation standard that values diversity and inclusion as core values to foster humanistic environments, it is not clear that dental schools have climates that are inclusive of minoritized people, whether they are patients, students, staff members or faculty members.[5,6] For the profession to advance oral health equity, intentional efforts for diverse people are essential.

[a] University of Maryland School of Dentistry, 650 West Baltimore Street, Baltimore, MD 21201-1586, USA; [b] Rutgers School of Dental Medicine, 110 Bergen Street, Room B-828, Newark, NJ 07101, USA
* Corresponding author.
E-mail address: efleming@umaryland.edu

Dent Clin N Am 69 (2025) 69–82
https://doi.org/10.1016/j.cden.2024.08.003   **dental.theclinics.com**

Historical Perspective

The issue of inclusion in dentistry is not a new concern. In 1866, the American Dental Association (ADA) adopted the first Code of Ethics, which emphasized the importance of prioritizing patients' needs while upholding ethical conduct in dentists' professional responsibilities. Since then, the ADA Principles of Ethics and Code of Conduct have evolved over the years.[7] Although some words such as diversity, equity, inclusion, and belonging (DEIB) are not explicitly presented, they are part of these principles. The relationship between the dental code of ethics and inclusion is one that, at its core, outlines the professional responsibilities and moral obligations of dental practitioners toward their patients, colleagues, and society at large. Inclusion, within the context of dentistry, can be defined as one that creates an environment where all individuals, regardless of their background, identity, or ability, feel valued, respected, and provided with equitable access to dental care. To highlight inclusivity in this important document, the principle of justice fosters and encourages dentists to be fair in their dealings and practice of dentistry for the benefit of all, while improving access to care to the community at large. Overall, the principles of the code of ethics intertwine with inclusivity, which promotes patient-centered care and upholds the values of respect, equity, and dignity within the dental profession. By embracing the principles of inclusion, dental professionals can ensure that their practices are not only ethically sound but also truly welcoming and accessible to all individuals in need of dental care.

In 1926, Dr. William J. Gies, who is considered the founder of modern dental education, published *Dental Education in the United States and Canada: A Report to the Carnegie Foundation for the Advancement of Teaching*.[8] In the report, Dr. Gies identified three fundamental areas that are essential for improving oral health: practice, education, and research.[8] While not a direct theme in Gies' writing, these areas are inclusive components currently. Gies indicated that the right dental education should include a cultural background for the dentist as for the physician (See two quotes selected from the Gies Report in **Box 1**).[8]

Looking back at this report, the exploration of dentistry from a historic lens allows for contemporary oral health professionals to better understand challenges to enhance diversity and inclusion in the profession of dentistry. Gies identified the need for a more significant number and more effective distribution of Black practitioners in the dental and medical professions.[8] Furthermore, Gies advocated for Black practitioners to participate and be integrated in the community for the welfare of the underrepresented population (see **Box 1**).[8]

Gies effectively argues for greater diversity in the oral health workforce to support the delivery of care to underserved populations, which is a cornerstone of health equity. Moreover, in naming the "economic, social, and educational conditions" (see **Box 1**)[8] that have been barriers to Black people for entering the profession, contemporary oral health professionals can glean from Gies that the profession has not lived up to being a humanistic environment inclusive of all people who want to be a part of the oral health team and, by extension, patients who may need care. Now is the time to explore how dentistry can become inclusive and embrace inclusion in its clinical practice and the recruitment and recruitment of the workforce that the 21st century requires.

Is 21st Century Dentistry Inclusive?

The U.S. is an increasingly diverse country.[9] At the 2020, Census the three most prevalent racial/ethnic groups in the United States are non-Hispanic White, Hispanic or

> **Box 1**
> **Two selected quotes pertinent to today from the 1926 Gies report[8]**
>
> *Education*
>   *The proper training of the practitioner is a matter of prime importance. That he should be an educated man, with a background of culture and refinement, is quite as essential for the dentist as for the physician. That his professional training should give him a true medical comprehension of his duties, as well as mechanical facility and esthetic felicity in the execution of his procedures, is equally obvious. In educational quality and influence, dental schools should equal medical schools, for their responsibilities are similar and their tasks are analogous. The dental graduate should be the peer of the medical graduate in all important personal attributes, and in professional capability. (Page 237)*
>
> *Need for Additional Dental Schools for Negroes*
>   *Economic, social, and educational conditions long conspired to prevent Negroes from entering the professions of health service. With improvement in the economic status of the colored group, however, the ability of Negroes to meet the expenses of a professional education is steadily growing. Inasmuch as prevailing sentiment for segregation prevents admission of more than a few colored students to the existing medical and dental schools attended by white students, there is evident need not only for improvement and support of such schools as are devoted exclusively to the training of Negroes, but also for an increase in their number. The creation of departments or schools for the training of Negroes in health service, in state universities or in universities having adequate endowments, should appeal strongly to the citizens of states containing large colored populations. (Page 93)*

Latino, and non-Hispanic Black.[9] The demographics of the United States are projected to continue to evolve with the country becoming minority White in 2045.[10] Given these changes in the country, questions arise as to how inclusive and diverse is the health care workforce for insuring health equity.[11] **Fig. 1** provides percentage contrasts of recent demographic data from the US populations to NIDCR grant applicants showing inconsistencies in representation.[12–14]

Is Dentistry a Humanistic Environment?

Minoritized populations in the United States, such as Black, Hispanic, American Indian/Alaska Native, Native Hawaiian and other Pacific Islanders, are underrepresented

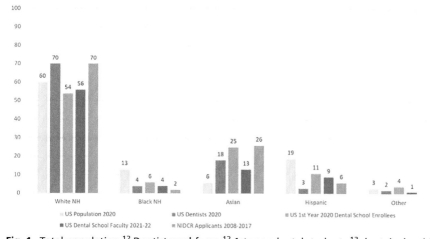

Fig. 1. Total population,[12] Dentist workforce,[12] 1st year dental students,[13] dental school faculty members,[13] and NIDCR extramural funding applicants[14] circa 2020 by race/ethnicity.

across various facets of the oral health workforce in corresponding proportions of these populations in the US population. While not expecting perfect parity in the workforce reflecting the population, it is telling that the disparities in the representation of minoritized population are so stark. Given a variety of reasons for the low level of diversity in dentistry, the question arises about whether dentistry is a humanistic environment.

The Commission on Dental Accreditation (CODA) emphasizes that inclusion should be evaluated as part of institutional climate in the accreditation process.[15] Institutional climate includes programs and initiatives established by the institution to actively support diversity as a fundamental value, creating an inclusive, engaging environment conducive to learning and professional growth for all. Recognizing diversity as crucial for academic excellence, CODA underscores the importance of dental schools creating environments that facilitate the exchange of ideas and beliefs across gender, racial, ethnic, cultural, and socio-economic backgrounds.[15] Hence, all dental schools are expected to support a humanistic, inclusive culture.[16]

The climate of dental schools

In 2022, the American Dental Education Association (ADEA) launched the first-ever climate study among dental schools and dental education programs in the United States and Canada. Preliminary by-variate findings were reported in November 2022.[17] Participants from 66 dental schools (88% of the dental schools) participated in the survey with an estimated overall response rate for participants from US Dental Schools of about 24%. Assessments included five composite scores for well-being, sense of belong, inclusive environment, inclusive culture, and welcomeness. See **Fig. 2** for US Dental Schools mean scores by Race/Ethnicity and Public versus Private Dental Schools.[17] Variations across these domains appear evident for different perceptions by respondents by the race/ethnicity groups. Nevertheless, the highest composite scores in the areas assessed were for welcomeness and the lowest were for inclusive environment. The mean scores for Private Dental Schools appear higher than those for Public Dental Schools or for all race/ethnicity groups, raising questions about the intersectionality issues that might be contained.

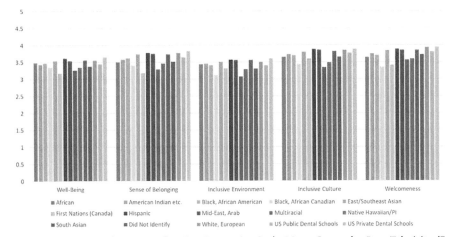

Fig. 2. 2022 ADEA Climate Study: Five Composite Scale Mean Scores by Race/Ethnicity (5-point Likert-Scale with range 1 = Strongly Disagree to 5 = Strongly Agree).[17]

Student experiences with discrimination

Few studies assess student experiences with discrimination in dentistry. As individual assessments were made regarding equitable policies and practices, cultural "competence", and harassment and discrimination in the 2022 ADEA Climate Survey.[17] (For a little insight, see **Box 2**). A qualitative study, using focus groups at a UK dental school in December 2020, found students in dental schools experience a range of racist encounters from stereotyping and microaggression to racial mocking.[18] In another qualitative study, using focus groups of minoritized dental students at a US school in spring 2021, students described experiences of discrimination trackable from their pre-dental training across applying to dental school and exploring career opportunities with post-graduate training.[19] Several studies at dental schools in the US surveyed students.[20,21] In the fall of 2011, one school's assessment, where 95% of the respondents were Hispanic or Black, 22% of students reported having experienced discrimination.[20] Another school survey using a discrimination questionnaire found Black/African Americans students scored the highest, and that all the non-White racial/ethnic groups had a higher mean score of perceived discrimination compared to the non-Hispanic White group of students.[21]

Dentists experiences with discrimination

A limited scholarship on the prevalence of discrimination in the dental workforce exists, particularly when focusing on race/ethnicity. Two studies provide context for questioning the degree to which dentistry embraces inclusion.[22,23] In an undated national assessment published in 2017, using 41 Black Oral and Maxillofacial Surgeons respondents to a survey distributed from the mailing list of the National Society of Oral and Maxillofacial Surgeons, 24% reported experiencing race-related harassment in their residencies, 54% perceived bias against African Americans in Oral and Maxillofacial Surgery residencies and 46% reported race-related harassment in their workplace.[22] In a 2012 national survey of underrepresented minority dentists, 72% of surveyed dentists reported any experience with discrimination in a dental setting,

---

Box 2
Select findings from the 2022 ADEA climate study for US Dental Schools[17]

Equitable Policies and Practices
• Experiences of Bias of Inequities
    With dress code, personal appearance, and attire: 26%
    With code of conduct or discipline policy: 26%
• Agree their dental school has effective strategic diversity goals and plans: 61%
• Agree their dental school has effective admissions practices and policies that increase student diversity: 63%
• Agree their dental school has effective hiring practices that increase faculty diversity: 55%
• Agree their dental school has effective hiring practices that increase staff diversity: 55%

Cultural Competence
• Agreed that since dental school, my understanding of the social determinants of health and how they impact oral health treatment has improved: 87% of US dental students

Harassment and Discrimination
• Experienced harassment in US Dental Schools: 13%
• Witnessed harassment in US Dental Schools: 20%
• Experienced discrimination in US Dental Schools: 17%
• Witnessed discrimination in US Dental Schools: 27%
• Experience harassment or discrimination in US Dental Schools: 34%

with the rates of experiences highest among Black dentists (86%) compared to 59% of Hispanic dentists and 49% American Indian/Alaska Native dentists.[23]

Patient experiences with discrimination

The first national study of discrimination experiences in oral care visits was conducted in 2022.[24] The existing Everyday Discrimination Scale was adapted to the oral care setting (EDSOC).[24] Minoritized survey respondents, specifically non-Hispanic Asian, non-Hispanic Black and Hispanic groups had higher mean scores on the discrimination scale than had the non-Hispanic White group of respondents.[24] Moreover, respondents with experiences of discrimination were associated with reporting fair/poor oral health, not having visited a dentist in Two years, and not planning a future oral care visit.[24] The study suggests that patient experiences with discrimination (ie, the lack of inclusivity in dentistry) may exacerbate oral health inequities.

A recent dissertation explored psychosocial and behavioral factors related to experiences with discrimination in oral health care settings for 751 Black adults' (ages 21–64 years) in Baltimore.[25] A concerning level of discrimination in oral health care settings is shown, with approximately half of the study participants indicating experiences of discrimination, which appears intensified if using emergency room serices.[25]

Challenges to Humanism and Inclusion

Debunking the myth of inclusion: "I don't see color"

"I don't see color" is a phrase that has been used for thinking that it deescalates tensions circa equity, diversity, and inclusion efforts. However, the underlying notion in the phase "I don't see color" is colorblindness.[26] Scholars argue that colorblindness becomes either a form of color evasion ("not seeing color") or power evasion (denying racism).[26–28] While colorblindness sounds harmless and inviting of a notion of "post-racial America", the phrase "I don't see color" actually serves as an affront to inclusion and efforts to advance justice.[29]

For minoritized, people of color who are told "I don't see color" may take the message as they are not seen: "I don't see color" can be understood as "You don't see me". The impact of these words can foster a sense of "othering" (the act of treating someone as though they are not part of a group and are different in some way[30]) and potentially cultivate imposter syndrome in minoritized people. Further, the process of "othering", students being particularly vulnerable, therefore poses a threat to the sense of inclusion and belonging that every dental school aspires to foster as a humanistic environment. For students who feel othered and forced to "blend in", they may experience imposter syndrome (UK "impostor"). Imposter syndrome "describes high-achieving individuals who, despite their objective successes, fail to internalize their accomplishments and have persistent self-doubt and fear of being exposed as a fraud or impostor."[31,32] For people experiencing imposter syndrome, they may "attribute successes to external factors such as luck or receiving help from others and attribute setbacks as evidence of their professional inadequacy".[31,33] In a systematic review, imposter syndrome was found "common among African American, Asian American, and Latino/a American college students and that imposter feelings are significantly negatively correlated with psychological well-being and positively correlated with depression and anxiety".[31] While no studies assessed the prevalence or impact of imposter syndrome among minoritized dental students, it is worth considering that the negative correlations with well-being among college students would be similar in professional students. Moreover, the feelings of imposter syndrome and othering can be imagined to be additive to negatively impact one's sense of belonging and inclusion at a dental school.

In the clinical setting, "othering" is a threat to trust and the delivery of optimal care. "Othering" spotlights the "social gulf," a term used by Otto to express differences between the oral health provider and patients.[34] Furthermore, the "social gulf" exacerbates power imbalances that can exist between the oral health provider and patients.[34] The lived experiences and social identities of the providers and patients creates an imbalance of power where the providers having specialized knowledge about oral health and clinical practice and perhaps lacking the knowledge and information about communities, social histories, and lived experiences may perceive patient behavior as "undesirable" or "deviant".[34] These negative perceptions and othering create a tension where the patient's ability to be heard and to trust the providers are threatened.[24]

"Inclusion Health": Re-Imagining Dentistry as an Inclusive Profession to Advance Health Equity

Inclusion is especially key in the health care professions as practitioners and leaders grapple with improving access to health care and improving health outcomes. A growing science and literature from the United Kingdom support the notion of "inclusion health".[35] "Inclusion health" centers social exclusion and populations made vulnerable by their social conditions, inviting health care provider, researchers, policy advocates, and other leaders to explore social exclusion as a driver of health outcomes.[35,36] The term "Inclusion Oral Health" emerged with the aim of the profession of dentistry to act as an agent of social inclusion as a solution to address oral health inequities globally (**Box 3**).[37] An application to dentistry focused on "inclusion health" can be seen in a recent paper by Bradley and colleagues on models of dental care for people experiencing homelessness.[38]

In these applications of inclusion in health and oral health, the effort is to move inclusion from beyond a buzzword and to offer inclusion as a praxis that includes research, policy, and practice agenda. Specifically, "inclusion oral health" offers a unique opportunity for dentistry and oral health professionals to tackle "othering" and foster trust and belonging as it relates to addressing oral health disparities.

Respectful Inclusion and Belonging

In creating a dental academic environment that supports inclusivity, efforts can be made to move beyond inclusivity to embrace the concept of "respectful inclusion".[39] "Respectful inclusion" is defined as establishing an environment where all individuals within an organization or institution are genuinely respected, valued, and seamlessly integrated into its culture.[39] This concept is particularly crucial in health profession

---

Box 3
Additional insight into inclusion oral health

Inclusion oral health is based on a theoretically engaged understanding on how social exclusion is produced and experienced, and how forms of exclusion and discrimination intersect to compound oral health outcomes. Inclusion oral health focuses on developing innovative inter-sectoral solutions to tackle the inequities of people enduring extreme oral health.[37]

When such social interactions have an 'us versus them mentality,' that is, between dental professionals and people who already are experiencing social exclusion, this dynamic can give rise to 'othering'. Othering is conceptualized as having three parts, which together create a social chasm: [a] making judgements about the other; [b] isolating the other; and [c] misunderstanding the other.[37]

education where both respectful inclusion and diversity are fundamental. They not only enhance learning and well-being among students but also contribute to preparing a health care workforce capable of addressing health disparities and advancing scientific understanding to meet societal needs.

Belonging as part of the respectful inclusion dynamic is important for advancing the concept. In 2023, the US Surgeon General's Advisory on the Healing Effects of Social Connection and Community report *Our Epidemic of Loneliness and Isolation*[40] spans multiple disciplines to stress the crucial role of social connection in individual health and community-wide metrics of health and well-being. The report defined "belonging" as a *fundamental human need, the feeling of deep connection with social groups, physical places, and individual and collective experiences.*[40] Notably, the degree of belonging can be significantly influenced by the perceived value of diversity within an organization, the perspectives of its leadership, and the efficacy of its policies. Each of these areas can lead to developing strategies to promote best practices to increase the sense of belonging.

Call to Action

Realizing humanism in dental education

Founded in 1923 as the American Association of Dental Schools,[41] ADEA has evolved into the leading advocate for dental education. In its commitment to fostering a diverse dental community ADEA has developed a significant array of resources that are invaluable to all members of the dental profession. The ADEA/W.K. Kellogg Foundation Minority Dental Faculty and Inclusion Program is a best practice on how to leverage a structured mentoring program to support minoritized faculty in their career and professional development.[42,43] The program utilized a framework that emphasizes diversity as a core value essential to enhancing the academic environment's quality for all students. By integrating the diversity of faculty across policies and programs, a mentoring program like this one can cultivate a more inclusive educational landscape.

In 2020, *The ADEA Faculty Diversity Toolkit* was developed to help address low faculty diversity in dental education.[44] This comprehensive document serves as a guide for dental schools and allied dental programs, offering best practices to recruit and retain historically underrepresented and marginalized faculty members. It provides strategic insights and resources to support institutions in fostering a diverse faculty body. Moreover, the toolkit highlights the significant barriers that dental schools can create for recruiting and retaining faculty.

Dental schools are not humanistic environments when people experience a lack of respect and consideration, an insufficient sense of community or belonging, and an institution with ineffective communication and a lack of support or inequitable access to professional development opportunities.[44] Additionally, the report advocates for "microaffirmations"[45] which are "small acts that foster inclusion, listening, comfort and support for people who may feel isolated or invisible in an environment that can be applied to challenging and affirming experiences.[44,45]

In 2022, *The Journal of Dental Education* published a Special Issue focusing on Diversity, Equity, Inclusion, and Belonging.[46] This issue contains a compilation of 23 articles addressing current challenges in dental education and proposing actionable strategies for fostering significant change. A platform is provided to drive conversations and initiatives aimed at advancing diversity, equity, inclusion, and a sense of belonging within the dental community. The Special Issue editors are clear that "our collective efforts will be required to create more inclusive, humanistic, accessible, and equitable environments throughout dental education where each person thrives, feels a strong connection, and has a sense of belonging.[47]"

In addition to these publications, ADEA actively supports and educates admission officers via implementing a Holistic Admission & Review process.[48] This initiative aims to assist dental schools in evaluating candidates as multifaceted individuals, considering their diverse competencies and experiences. By acknowledging selection bias in admissions, dental schools that practice holistic admissions can ensure that their admissions policies and practices support humanism and inclusive culture for students.[49]

ADEA's commitment to promoting diversity and equity within dental education and practice is evident through these resources, which provide essential tools and insights to advance inclusive practices across the profession. Since its inception, ADEA has prioritized diversity, equity, and inclusion in dental education, continually striving to cultivate an environment that embraces individuals from all backgrounds.[50] This ongoing dedication ensures equal opportunities for advancement and success within the dental profession (**Boxes 4** and **5**) provides a summary of guidance for consideration by dental education.

Leveraging inclusion to advance health equity

Inclusion is a central component to advancing oral health equity,[37] and yet, inclusion alone will not realize health equity. The World Health Organization (WHO) defines health equity as: "the absence of unfair, avoidable and remediable differences in health status among groups of people."[51] WHO continues that "health equity is achieved when everyone can attain their full potential for health and well-being."[51] For inclusion to better align with health equity and to improve population-level health outcomes, consideration must be made of two facts: people and community.

For people and individual patients, inclusive practices include person-centered care practices: "Within a person-centered care environment, a person is a recipient of care, and can act as a partner who co-designs his/her care delivery."[52] The degree to which the voice of the individual patients informs their care is key for the advancement for oral health equity, specifically the removal of those barriers that impede the full potential for health.

At the community level, inclusion is paramount in the collection of data and in communication. Complete public health data require the inclusion of all communities, especially those who bear the disproportionate burden of disease. In public health data systems, often data are limited for certain minoritized groups, such as American Indian and Alaska Native people, Asian American and Pacific Islanders, and Native Hawaiian and Pacific Islanders, and sexual and gender minorities. Incomplete data are problematic as minoritized groups find themselves categorized as "other" due

---

Box 4
Dental school care points based on ADEA policy[50]

- Dental schools should leverage humanism to advance an environment of respectful inclusion.

- A diverse faculty body is key to supporting an inclusive environment for students, staff, and other faculty.

- Evaluating and enhancing the admissions processes on diversity with reflection on the patient population should be an approach made by dental schools.

- Dental schools should follow the outlined practices from the American Dental Education Association to support a more inclusive culture.

Box 5
Call to action

To reimagine dentistry as a respectful and inclusive profession that not only values diversity but also harnesses its transformative potential through intentional inclusion, several key recommendations are essential to propel the profession into the 21st century.

- Historical Perspective: Understanding the history of the dental profession reveals minimal progress in diversity. This historical context should prompt leaders in the field to prioritize advancing diversity for the profession's long-term benefit.
- Commission on Dental Accreditation (CODA) Standards: While CODA standards emphasize diversity as pivotal for nurturing humanistic environments, it remains unclear if dental schools provide inclusive climates for minoritized individuals—whether as students or faculty. Dental school leaders should underscore these standards to stakeholders, enhancing awareness of their evaluation criteria and emphasizing the institutional commitment to diversity and inclusive respect.
- ADEA Resources: Familiarizing oneself with the wealth of resources offered by the American Dental Education Association (ADEA) and other agencies supporting dental education is crucial.
- Best Practices: To identify other dental schools as well as health care institutions with innovative practices in fostering an environment where diversity, equity, respectful inclusion and belonging are valued.

---

to the small numbers in the sample.[53–56] Complete data that allow for all social demographics are key for improving population-level health. In national oral health data, these previously named groups are often excluded with limited data describing oral health outcomes except for reports from the Indian Health Service. The lack of inclusion exacerbates health disparities.

Inclusive communication is also key for advancing health equity. Inclusive communication is more than language that meets 508 compliance standards.[57,58] Inclusive communication must be accessible for people with disabilities and allow for culturally appropriate images, the use of preferred terms, and language that is people-centered. Inclusive communication in the form of people-centered language is critical for care delivery. In contrast to a traditional, medical model of communication that focuses on a patient's diagnosis and takes a paternalistic approach of reassuring patients rather than engaging them as decision-makers in their care, people-centered care with inclusive language allows for "treating patients as partners, involving them in planning their health care and encouraging them to take responsibility for their own health."[57]

In a care-delivery setting, using person-centered language centers the individual and not their diagnosis or condition. Person-centered language takes as foundational understanding that individuals are the experts on their lives and health.[59] Examples include: "person with oral cancer," "person with a substance use disorder," and "person with a disability."[60] Inclusion communication requires respect for an individual's language preference and using preferred gender pronouns. In humanizing people, inclusive communication can also center strength-based language. Strength-based language, as opposed to deficit-based language, invites less negative bias in working with patients.[60]

SUMMARY

Inclusion has important implications for the practice of dentistry and how dental schools function and support the diverse workforce that is needed to advance oral health equity. Inclusion is more than maintaining a diversity of people but must foster belonging in institutions and in clinical practices. For inclusion to support belonging, there must be a leadership focus and the implication of policies to support best practices. In terms of clinical practices, people-centered and equity-focused communication can support the dental professional ethic of justice and include the patient as an active participant in their care. The absence of inclusion and belonging fosters settings that are unsafe for leaders, practitioners, learners, and patients. Oral professional should aim to create more safe spaces for learning and care delivery.

CLINICS CARE POINTS

- To create a patient-centered care environment and a student-centered learning environment, dentistry should embrace inclusion and apply practices that foster belonging.
- Adhere to the profession's ethical principles and code of conduct to cultivate an environment that is fair, respectful, and safe for everyone.
- Inclusive communication strategies and practices are essential in clinical practice.
- Inclusive language allows for everyone to be treated as partners in their health care delivery and in learning.

DISCLOSURE

The authors have nothing to disclose.

REFERENCES

1. Garcia RI, Blue Spruce G, Sinkford JC, et al. Workforce diversity in dentistry - current status and future challenges. J Publ Health Dent 2017;77(2):99–104.
2. Majerczyk D, Behnen EM, Weldon DJ, et al. Racial, ethnic, and sex diversity trends in health professions programs from applicants to graduates. JAMA Netw Open 2023;6(12):e2347817.
3. Nasseh K, Fosse C, Vujicic M. Dentists who participate in medicaid: who they are, where they locate, how they practice. Med Care Res Rev 2023;80(2):245–52.
4. Mertz EA, Wides CD, Kottek AM, et al. Underrepresented minority dentists: quantifying their numbers and characterizing the communities they serve. Health Aff (Millwood) 2016;35(12):2190–9.
5. Smith PD, Evans CA, Fleming E, et al. Establishing an antiracism framework for dental education through critical assessment of accreditation standards. J Dent Educ 2022;86(9):1063–74.
6. Fleming E, Smith CS, Ware TK, et al. Can academic dentistry become an antiracist institution? Addressing racial battle fatigue and building belonging. J Dent Educ 2022;86(9):1075–82.
7. American Dental Association. Principles of ethics and code of conduct. 2023. Available at: https://www.ada.org/-/media/project/ada-organization/ada/ada-org/files/about/ada_code_of_ethics.pdf?rev=ba22edfdf1a646be9249fe2d870d7d31&hash=CCD76FCDC56D6F2CCBC46F1751F51B96. Accessed July 4, 2024.
8. Gies WJ. Dental education in the United States and Canada: a report to the Carnegie Foundation for the advancement of teaching. Boston: DB Updike Merrymount Press; 1926. Available at: http://archive.carnegiefoundation.org/publications/pdfs/elibrary/Gies_Report.pdf. Accessed July 10, 2024.

9. Jensen E, Jones N, Rabe M, et al. The chance that two people chosen at random are of different race or ethnicity groups has increased since 2010. 2021. Available at: https://www.census.gov/library/stories/2021/08/2020-united-states-population-more-racially-ethnically-diverse-than-2010.html. Accessed July 4, 2024.

10. Frey WH. Diversity explosion: how new racial demographics are remaking America. Washington, DC: The Brookings Institution; 2018.

11. Pittman P, Chen C, Erikson C, et al. Health workforce for health equity. Med Care 2021;59(Suppl 5):S405–8.

12. American Dental Association. U.S. Dentist demographics dashboard. Available at: https://www.ada.org/resources/research/health-policy-institute/us-dentist-demographics https://www.ada.org/resources/research/health-policy-institute/dentist-workforce https://www.ada.org/resources/research/health-policy-institute/dental-education. Accessed July 4, 2024.

13. American Dental Education Association. ADEA 2023-24 trends in dental education. Available at: https://www.adea.org/DentEdTrends/. Accessed July 4, 2024.

14. National Institute of Dental and Craniofacial Research. NIDCR strategic plan 2021-2026. Available at: https://www.nidcr.nih.gov/sites/default/files/2022-01/NIDCR-Strategic-Plan-2021-2026.pdf. Accessed July 1, 2024.

15. Commission on Dental Accreditation. Commission on dental accreditation standards for dental education programs. 2023. Available at: https://coda.ada.org/. Accessed July 4, 2024.

16. Lyon L, Itaya LE, Hoover T, et al. Humanism in dental education: a comparison of theory, intention, and stakeholder perceptions at a north American dental school. J Dent Educ 2017;81(8):929–36.

17. American Dental Education Association, 2022 ADEA climate study: overview of preliminary key findings and data, Available at: https://www.adea.org/ClimateStudy/Key-Findings/. (Accessed September 3 2024), 2023.

18. Ahmadifard A, Forouhi S, Waterhouse P, et al. A student-led qualitative study to explore dental undergraduates' understanding, experiences, and responses to racism in a dental school. J Publ Health Dent 2022;82(S1):36–45.

19. Fleming E, Agyemfra M, Anige N, et al. Building sustainable approaches to recruit, retain, and professionalize Black, Latinx, and American Indian students interested in dental careers. J Dent Educ 2022;86(9):1090–7.

20. McCann AL, Lacy ES, Miller BH. Underrepresented minority students' experiences at Baylor College of Dentistry: perceptions of cultural climate and reasons for choosing to attend. J Dent Educ 2014;78(3):411–22.

21. Akinkugbe AA, Raskin SE, Garcia DT. Heightened vigilance and perceived discrimination in dental trainees' readiness for clinical practice. J Dent Educ 2023;87(8):1123–32.

22. Criddle TR, Gordon NC, Blakey G, et al. African Americans in oral and maxillofacial Surgery: factors affecting career choice, satisfaction, and practice patterns. J Oral Maxillofac Surg 2017;75(12):2489–96.

23. Fleming E, Mertz E, Jura M, et al. American Indian/Alaska Native, Black, and Hispanic dentists' experiences of discrimination. J Publ Health Dent 2022;82(Suppl 1):46–52.

24. Raskin SE, Thakkar-Samtani M, Santoro M, et al. Discrimination and dignity experiences in prior oral care visits predict racialized oral health inequities among nationally representative US adults. J Racial Ethn Health Disparities 2023. https://doi.org/10.1007/s40615-023-01821-0.

25. Phillips B. Intersectionality, racial discrimination and oral healthcare utilization among Black adults in Baltimore city, Maryland [doctoral dissertation, Virginia

commonwealth university]. 2024. Available at: https://scholarscompass.vcu.edu/etd/7753/. Accessed May 7, 2026.

26. Mekawi Y, Todd NR, Yi J, et al. Distinguishing "I don't see color" from "Racism is a thing of the past": psychological correlates of avoiding race and denying racism. J Counsel Psychol 2020;67(3):288–302.

27. Neville HA, Gallardo ME, Sue DW, editors. The myth of racial color blindness. Washington, DC: American Psychological Association; 2016.

28. Neville HA, Awad GH, Brooks JE, et al. Color-blind racial ideology: theory, training, and measurement implications in psychology. Am Psychol 2013;68(6): 455–66.

29. Daughtry KA, Earnshaw V, Palkovitz R, et al. You blind? What, you can't see that? The impact of colorblind attitude on young adults' activist behavior against racial injustice and racism in the U.S. J Afr Am Stud 2020;24(1):1–22.

30. Cambridge Dictionary. Definition of othering. Available at: https://dictionary.cambridge.org/us/dictionary/english/othering. Accessed July 10, 2024.

31. Bravata DM, Watts SA, Keefer AL, et al. Prevalence, predictors, and treatment of impostor syndrome: a systematic review. J Gen Intern Med 2020;35(4):1252–75.

32. Kolligian J, Sternberg RJ. Perceived fraudulence in young adults: is there an "imposter syndrome"? J Pers Assess 1991;56(2):308–26.

33. Clance PR, Imes SA. The imposter phenomenon in high achieving women: dynamics and therapeutic intervention. Psychother Theory Res Pract 1978;15(3): 241–7.

34. Otto OM. Teeth: the story of beauty, inequality, and the struggle for oral health in America. New York, (NY): The New Press; 2016.

35. Luchenski S, Maguire N, Aldridge RW, et al. What works in inclusion health: overview of effective interventions for marginalised and excluded populations. Lancet 2018;391:266–80.

36. Marmot M. Inclusion health: addressing the causes of the causes. Lancet 2018; 391(10117):186–8.

37. Freeman R, Doughty J, Macdonald ME, et al. Inclusion oral health: advancing a theoretical framework for policy, research and practice. Community Dent Oral Epidemiol 2020;48(1):1–6.

38. Bradley N, Heidari E, Andreasson S, et al. Models of dental care for people experiencing homelessness in the UK: a scoping review of the literature. Br Dent J 2023;234(11):816–24.

39. Roberts LW. Belonging, respectful inclusion, and diversity in medical education. Acad Med 2020;95(5):661–4.

40. Office of the Surgeon General (OSG). Our Epidemic of Loneliness and Isolation: The U.S. Surgeon General's Advisory on the Healing Effects of Social Connection and Community. Washington (DC): US Department of Health and Human Services; 2023.

41. American Dental Education Association. ADEA celebrates 100 years. Available at: https://www.adea.org/Press/Jan2023-ADEA-Celebrates-100-Years/. Accessed July 15, 2014.

42. Beech BM, Calles-Escandon J, Hairston KG, et al. Mentoring programs for under-represented minority faculty in academic medical centers: a systematic review of the literature. Acad Med 2013;88(4):541–9.

43. Sinkford JC, West JF, Weaver RG, et al. Modelling mentoring: early lessons from the W.K. Kellogg/ADEA minority dental faculty development program. J Dent Educ 2009;73:753–63.

44. Smith S, Lee A, Gilbert J. ADEA faculty diversity toolkit. Washington, DC: American Dental Education Association; 2020.
45. Rowe M. Micro-affirmations and microinequities. J International Ombudsman Association 2008;1(1):45–8.
46. Issue information. Special Issue of the Journal of Dental Education September 2022. J Dent Educ 2022;86(9):1047–50.
47. Sinkford JC, Smith SG. Introduction to this special issue. J Dent Educ 2022;86: 1051–4.
48. Booker C, Rhineberger E, Lowery L. Holistic admissions in dental education 2022 and beyond. J Dent Educ 2022;86:1107–12.
49. Chaviano-Moran R, Chuck E, Perez H. Unintended demographic bias in GPA/ DAT-Based pre-admission screening: an argument for holistic admissions in dental schools. J Dent Educ 2019;83(11):1280–8.
50. ADEA. Statement of ADEA policy on diversity and inclusion. Available at: https://www. adea.org/policy_advocacy/diversity_equity/pages/diversityandinclusion.aspx#. Accessed July 15, 2024.
51. World Health Organization. Health equity and its determinants. World Health Day 2021: it's time to build a fairer, healthier world for everyone, everywhere. Geneva: World Health Organization; 2021. Available at: https://cdn.who.int/media/docs/ default-source/world-health-day-2021/health-equity-and-its-determinants.pdf. Accessed July 11, 2024.
52. Lee H, Chalmers NI, Brow A, et al. Person-centered care model in dentistry. BMC Oral Health 2018;18(1):198.
53. Pete D, Erickson SL, Jim MA, et al. COVID-19 among non-hispanic American Indian and Alaska native people residing in urban areas before and after vaccine rollout-selected states and counties, United States, January 2020-October 2021. Am J Publ Health 2022;112(10):1489–97.
54. American Medical Association. AAPI community data needed to assess better health outcomes. 2020. Available at: https://www.ama-assn.org/system/files/ 2020-05/che-aapi-data-report.pdf. Accessed July 11, 2024.
55. Morey BN, Penaia CS, Tulua A, et al. Democratizing native Hawaiian and pacific islander data: examining community accessibility of data for health and the social drivers of health. Am J Publ Health 2024;114(S1):S103–11.
56. Patterson JG, Jabson JM, Bowen DJ. Measuring sexual and gender minority populations in health surveillance. LGBT Health 2017;4(2):82–105.
57. Kumar R, Chattu VK. What is in the name? Understanding terminologies of patient-centered, person-centered, and patient-directed care. J Fam Med Prim Care 2018;7(3):487–8.
58. Calanan RM, Bonds ME, Bedrosian SR, et al. CDC's guiding principles to promote an equity-centered approach to public health communication. Prev Chronic Dis 2023;20:E57.
59. Americans with Disabilities Act National Network. Guidelines for writing about people with disabilities. 2018. Available at: https://adata.org/factsheet/ADANN-writing.html. Accessed July 4, 2024.
60. Hyams K, Prater N, Rohovit J, et al. Person-centered Language. Clinical Tip No. 8 (April, 2018): St. Paul: Minnesota Center for Chemical and Mental Health, University of Minnesota. https://practicetransformation.umn.edu/wp-content/uploads/ 2019/01/9.-MNCAMH-Clinical-Tip-Person-Centered-Language-May-11-2018.pdf. Accessed September 9, 2024.

United States Dental School Deans' Characteristics Through an Inclusive Lens

Linda M. Kaste, DDS, MS, PhD, FAADOCR, FICD[a],*,
Judy Chia-Chun Yuan, DDS, MS, MAS[b]

KEYWORDS

- Dental schools • Dental education • Deans • Inclusion • Women • Men • Diversity
- United States

KEY POINTS

- Historic data indicate the gradually increasing diversity among dental school deans, and contrast with the April 2024 cohort being the most diverse yet.
- The April 2024 Cohort of the United States Dental School deans approaches or meets the critical mass benchmark of 30% representation on several critical facets.
- Nearly a quarter of these deans have received international dental training, enhancing diversity and inclusivity reflective of the evolving dental student and general populations.
- Ongoing challenges include the persistence of underrepresentation of historically underrepresented minorities.
- Data monitoring and leadership training initiatives are essential to ensure progress in diversity and inclusion with dental school leadership.

INTRODUCTION

The composition of the United States (US) is becoming increasingly diverse from a dental perspective whether looking at the patient population, students, practitioners, or leaders. Recent trends (2000 – 2020) on selected demographics (**Fig. 1**) show contrasts among the US population,[1] the dentist workforce,[2] first year dental students,[3,4] and US dental school deans.[5–7] Through an inclusive lens, this article examines the status of dental school deans amidst this evolving diversity.

Diversity in the dental workforce and its translation to dental education has been discussed for decades.[8] For some aspects, diversity and access have taken small steps for over a century (**Fig. 2**).[9–29] Becoming more diverse contrasts with a

[a] Department of Oral Biology, University of Illinois Chicago College of Dentistry, Chicago, IL, USA; [b] Department of Restorative Dentistry, University of Illinois Chicago College of Dentistry, Chicago, IL, USA
* Corresponding author. UIC COD Department of Oral Biology, MC 690, Chicago, IL 60612.
E-mail address: kaste@uic.edu

Dent Clin N Am 69 (2025) 83–101
https://doi.org/10.1016/j.cden.2024.08.004   dental.theclinics.com

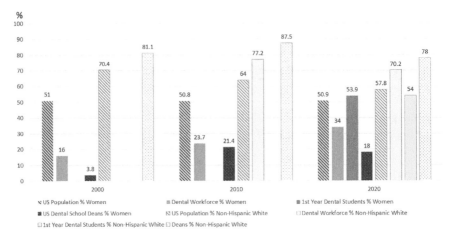

Fig. 1. Contrasts of the United States (US) Population, US Dental Workforce, US Dental 1st Year Dental Students, and US Dental school Deans by Percentages of Women and Non-Hispanic Whites (Circa 2000 – Circa 2020).[1–7]

considerable history of dental deans being predominantly White males.[6,30] Data for women versus men as the deans of US dental schools have been monitored, albeit with changing emphasis on terminology concerning sex and gender. These terms are examined in an accompanying chapter in this Dental Clinics of North American (DCNA) issue.[31] "Sex" refers to "female or male" for biologic characteristics and "gender" refers to "woman or man" for social characteristics. In this article with the focus on social characteristics, gender is used. Instead of using race/ethnicity, this article uses a modification of Culturally and Linguistically Diverse (CALD)[32,33] for a broad scope of sociocultural distinctions. Three categories of CALD are presented: (1) Non-Hispanic White/largely European American (White), (2) historically underrepresented minority (URM), concentrating on Black (African American is used in the paper when used by the original source) and Hispanic, but also would include Native American/American Indian or Alaskan Natives, and (3) other diverse groups (other CALD). Another element of observed diversity among US dental school deans is that of international dental school training (IDT).

To appreciate the historic context and advancements in diversity in US dental leadership, this article provides brief reviews of women and men, CALD, and IDT in dentistry and for dental school deans. Following those reviews, the current (April 2024) cohort of US dental school deans is assessed, and an overview of future contributions toward enhancing inclusivity is offered.

Women and Men

Lucy Beaman Hobbs Taylor, the first woman to graduate from a US dental school, completed her studies in 1866 from the Ohio College of Dental Surgery.[9] Between 1866 and 1893, 26.0% of the 181 women who graduated from US dental schools were foreign-born.[34] For a century, the number of women graduates remained low. However, between 1970 and 1984, the percentage of women entering dental school rose from 2% to 25%.[35,36] By 2001, women represented 40% of entering dental school classes[36] and in 2018, women surpassed the rate of men entering US dental schools.[37]

The first woman to be named as a dental school dean was Dr Jeanne Sinkford at Howard University in 1975,[20] whereas the first man to be named a US dental school

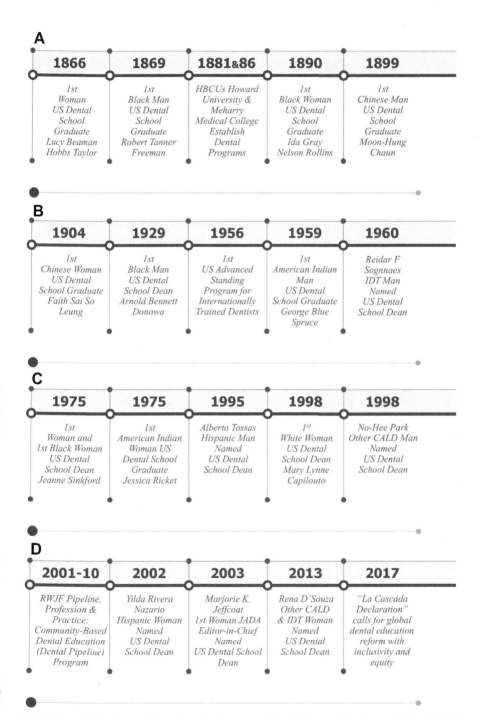

Fig. 2. Diversifying Steps of Dentistry leading toward Inclusion and the Current Cohort of US Dental School Deans [9–29] *(A) Sected Highlights 1860 - before 1900, (B) Selected Highlights 1900 - before 1975, (C) Selected Highlights 1975 - before 2000, and (D) Selected Highlights after 2000.*

dean was Dr Chapin A. Harris at the Baltimore College of Dental Surgery in 1840.[38] See **Box 1** for early pathfinder women who continued the movement that Dr Sinkford started.[20,23,26,27,39–44] Representation of women in dental faculty and leadership slowly grew,[7,45,46] such as during 2020 to 2021, women comprised 17.6% of the 68 US dental school deans.[7]

Historically, evidence supported that women meet higher standards than men to attain dental leadership positions.[47] A 2020 National Academies of Science review found ongoing challenges in the representation of women in academic leadership and recommended capturing the data to increase transparency.[48] Understanding these challenges is important for improving women's representation.[47,49] Leadership training directed at women in dentistry started in the 1990s.[50–52] American Dental Education Association (ADEA) initiated women's leadership development programs in 1992 with the Women Liaison Officer Group, followed by the Enid A Neidle Scholars Program in 1994, and support for the Hedwig van Ameringen Executive Leadership in Academic Medicine program at Drexel University in 1996.[51] From 1994 to 1999, ADEA offered a summer leadership program, later replaced with the ADEA Leadership Institute.[52] ADEA also created initiatives such as the Women in Leadership section and the Women Liaisons Officers to advance women and improve the academic environment for women on faculty.[53]

Contrasting high representation among dental students and faculty members, women remain underrepresented as deans of US dental schools. From 2000 to 2021 (**Fig. 3**), the proportion of women in these leadership positions rose.[5–7,54]

Culturally and Linguistically Diversity

CALD group members have been a part of the US dental workforce throughout its history. Focus on CALD inclusion in dental education has been primarily on Blacks. The first dental school, the Baltimore College of Dental Surgery, was founded in 1840 when an estimated 120 Blacks practiced dentistry in the US.[11]

Dr Robert Tanner Freeman faced rejection by two dental schools upon their recognition of his race but was admitted as one of the first six dental students to attend the Harvard University's School of Dental Medicine in 1867, adhering to the University's policy that it "would know no distinction of nativity or color".[10] Freeman graduated March 10, 1869, as the first degreed African American dentist in the US.[10,11] Harvard took over 100 years to graduate its first African American woman, Dr Dolores M Franklin, in 1974.[55]

In 1890, Dr Ida Gray Nelson Rollins was the first African American woman to graduate from a US dental school.[11,12] She worked in the dental office of Dr Jonathan Taft

Box 1			
Women early pioneers as the deans at United States dental schools[20,23,26,27,39–44]			
Jeanne Sinkford	1975	Howard University	Black
Eugenia Mobley	1978	Meharry Medical College	Black
Mary Lynne Capilouto	1998	University of Alabama	White
Sharon Turner	1998	Oregon Health & Science University	White
Cecile A. Feldman	2001	University of Medicine and Dentistry of New Jersey	White
Yilda Rivera Nazario	2002	University of Puerto Rico	Hispanic
Martha Somerman	2002	University of Washington	White
Terri A Dolan	2003	University of Florida	White
Connie Drisko	2003	Medical College of Georgia	White
Marjorie Jeffcoat	2003	University of Pennsylvania	White

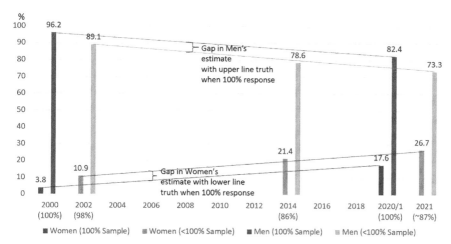

Fig. 3. United States (US) Dental School Deans' Representation by women and men between 2000 and 2021 showing contrasts between assessments with 100% representation and less than 100% representation (Response Rate).[5–7,54]

who was the first dean of the Dental College at the University of Michigan, which is thought to contribute to his advocating for her to become a dentist.[12]

Howard University and Meharry Medical College dental schools are the only dental schools of the 107 Historically Black Colleges and Universities (HBCU).[56] Howard's dental program was established around 1881 and Meharry's in 1886, both originally included in their respective medical schools.[11] The contributions of these schools to dental leadership and the proportion of the Black dentists are noteworthy. Dr Arnold Bennett Donowa, a Trinidad-born Howard graduate (Howard, 1922) became Howard's dean in 1929 and is considered the first US African American dental school dean, serving 2 years.[15] He was succeeded by Dr Russel Alexander Dixon (Northwestern, 1929) who served as Howard's dean from 1931 until 1966.[10,57] Dr Dixon influenced Dr Jeanne Sinkford (Howard, 1958) who in 1975 at Howard became the first woman and the first Black woman, to be the dean of a US dental school.[20]

By 2000, several men became first African American deans of non-HBCU dental schools.[58] These men included Dr Theodore E Bolden (Meharry, 1947) in 1977 at the now Rutgers dental school, Dr Frank M Lapeyrolerie (Howard, 1953) in 1979 at the now Rutgers dental school, Dr Raymond Fonseca (Connecticut, 1973) in 1989 at the University of Pennsylvania dental school, Dr Ronald Johnson (Pittsburgh, 1961) in 1994 at the now University of Texas Health Science Center at Houston dental school, and Dr Lonnie Norris (Harvard, 1976) in 1995 at Tufts dental school.[58]

In 1975, the same year that Dr Sinkford became the first woman US dental school dean, Dr Jessica Ricket graduated from the University of Michigan as the first American Indian woman dentist.[21] Dr George Blue Spruce, who obtained his Doctor of Dental Surgery in 1956 from Creighton University School of Dentistry, is the first American Indian dentist.[17] Approximately 50 years earlier, Dr Charles Goodall Lee[59] and Dr Faith Sai So Leong,[14] both of Chinese ancestry, graduated from the now University of the Pacific dental school, becoming the first Chinese American female and male dentists in the US.[14,59] The University of Pennsylvania dental school had an earlier Chinese graduate in 1899, Dr Moon-hung Chaun, although his career was in Hong Kong.[13] Dr No-Hee Park, possibly the first Asian-American dental school dean, served as dean of the University of California, Los Angeles (UCLA) School of Dentistry from 1998 to 2016.[24] Dr Rena D'Souza may be the first Asian/Indian woman dean when she became dean at the University of Utah in 2013.[28]

Information on the history of Hispanic dental education was first proved challenging to find. In 1997, Dr Alberto Tossas became the first alumnus of the University of Puerto Rico School of Dental Medicine to become its dean, possibly the first Hispanic dean of a US dental school.[22] In 2002, Dr Yilda Rivera Nazario was the first woman to take a similar path to dean.[26]

The designation as an HBCU is one example of institutional designations and histories. Another is Hispanic Serving Institutions (HSI), which have at least 25% Hispanic enrollment.[60] As of 2020 to 2021, 6 dental schools are at HSI designated universities.[61] Tribal Colleges and Universities (TCUs) is another institutional designation of history like HBCU; however, none of the 35 TCUs has a dental school.[62] Considering access as a part of inclusion, in 2001 15 dental schools began participation in a national demonstration program,[25] which showed impact on dental student experiences and characteristics.[63]

Dental schools and associated institutions have other aspects of interest possibly related to inclusivity and CALD. The missions and visions of schools reflect their histories and commitments. These aspects, not explored in this article, include religious salience[64] plausibly through dental schools being at institutions with religious affiliations such as Catholic/Jesuit, Jewish, Seventh Day Adventist, and United Methodist. Another example of institutional diversity is for dental schools associated with osteopathic medicine, which may have different cultural or philosophic commitments[65,66] than those associated with allopathic medicine, and which may differ from those having no medical or other health sciences affiliation.

International Dental Training

The US has long benefited from the contributions of leaders in dentistry who had received their training abroad, although detailed records among the firsts with IDT are scant. Notable examples (see **Fig. 2**) of such deans are Reidar F. Sognnaes, LDS, PhD, DMD, who first received dental education in Norway, served as the acting dean for Harvard (1959–1960) and was the founding dean for UCLA (1960–1968)[18,19] and Rena D'Souza, BDS, DMD, PhD who received her first dental training in India and was named the first woman dean at the University of Utah dental school in 2013.[28]

Having foreign trained dentists in the US, particularly related to US dental school faculty shortages, has been discussed for years with numerous pros and cons debated.[67–71] One concern voiced is "brain-drain" from Canada if positions in the US attract Canadian deans away.[70] Presence of IDT and general international influence can be seen in 4% of responses to a workforce survey in 1987[72] and for 5.7% of the 2020 to 2021 incoming US dental school dental students being from outside the US or Canada.[4]

Internationally trained dentists navigate various pathways to practice their profession and integrate into the workforce.[73] One of the primary pathways is through advanced standing programs associated with the ADEA Centralized Application for Advanced Placement for International Dentists[74], which allow IDT dentists to earn a US dental degree through an abbreviated training process. Tufts University School of Dental Medicine established one of the earliest such programs in 1956.[16] Currently, 42 US dental schools offer advanced programs for dentists with IDT.[75] Another pathway that IDT dentists can pursue is post-graduate training in various dental specialties, leading to eligibility for specialty licensure in the US.[73] Some states offer faculty licenses for IDT dentists to practice within academic institutions.[73]

Assessment of the April 2024 Dean Cohort

To assess current dean status, information is a census in April 2024 of the permanently named deans of US dental schools recognized by Commission on Dental Acceredition (CODA). The assessment uses publicly available information from dental-school websites and internet searches, as well as organized dentistry reports from the American Dental Association (ADA) and ADEA. This assessment is non-human subject research for use of publicly available information on these public figures in the context of their positions as dental school deans. The assessment was conducted similarly to other assessments[7] to avoid questionnaire low response rates by deans. **Fig. 3** provides an example of differences in estimates when using responses for deans' profiles versus 100% representation, where the questionnaire responses show overestimates of women as deans, as women were more likely to participate. Both modalities show increasing representation of women as deans.

The deans' personal characteristics identifiable from public use materials included basic demographics information such as photo and name recognition as woman or man; White, URM (Black or Hispanic only as none of the deans appeared to be of other recognized URM groups), or other CALD; education and training; and degrees beyond dental degrees, advanced education training, and associated board certification. Dental school characteristics where the deans hold their appointments include year of appointment, ADEA region, school funding designation (collapsed to 2 levels of public or private/private state-related), if the dean attended the school for training, and National Institute of Dental and Craniofacial Research (NIDCR) institutional grant funding ranking for 2023. Bivariate comparisons were conducted, focusing on similarities and distinctions between deans' characteristics distributions by gender, CALD category, and IDT.

The April 2024 United States Dental School Dean Cohort

Overall

This 2024 April Cohort assessment focuses on the 65 permanently named deans at the US dental schools recognized by CODA. See **Box 2** for basic dean demographics for the component groupings of dental school leading to this cohort.

Women versus men

Out of these 65 permanently named deans, the men-to-women ratio is approximately 2:1, with nearly 30% women (**Table 1**). On individual characteristics, this cohort of

Box 2			
Components leading to the April 2024 Dean Cohort of Permanent Deans at Commission on Dental Acceredition Recognized United States Dental Schools: Dean Demographics			
80 Dental Schools Existing or Proposed			
77 with Named Deans	31.2% Women	67.5% White	22.1% IDT
		14.3% URM	
		18.2% Other CALD	
9 Interim Deans	55.6% Women	55.6% White	22.2% IDT
		22.2% URM	
		22.2% Other CALD	
71 Accredited Schools	32.4% Women	67.6% White	23.9% IDT
		14.1% URM	
		18.3% Other CALD	
65 Accredited Schools with Permanent Deans	29.2% Women	69.2% White	23.1% IDT
		12.3% URM	
		18.5% Other CALD	

Table 1
Personal characteristics of the April 2024 cohort of permanently named deans at Commission on Dental Accreditation-recognized United States dental schools by gender, cultural, and linguistic diversity and dental degree location

Characteristic	Total	Gender		P-Value	Cultural and Linguistical Diversity			P-Value	Non-White P-Value	Dental Degree Location		P-Value
		Women	Men		White	URM	Other CALD			US Only	International (IDT)	
Total Counts (Row %)	65 (100%)	19 (29.2%)	46 (70.8%)	-	45 (69.2%)	8 (12.3%)	12 (18.5%)	-	-	50 (76.9%)	15 (23.1%)	-
Appointment Year Mean (SD)	2018.3 (4.9)	2018.8 (6.1)	2018.1 (4.4)	0.617	2018.4 (5.2)	2017.4 (3.4)	2018.4 (5.2)	0.854	0.741	2018.1 (5.0)	2019.1 (4.8)	0.502
Dental Graduation Year Mean (SD)	1987.0 (9.0)	1988.8 (8.3)	1986.2 (9.3)	0.290	1985.5 (8.3)	1984.5 (4.5)	1994.2 (10.5)	0.007	0.047	1986.0 (7.9)	1990.3 (11.8)	0.102
Years between Dental & Appointment Mean (SD)	32.3 (9.4)	30.0 (8.4)	31.9 (9.8)	0.451	32.9 (8.7)	32.9 (5.7)	24.3 (10.8)	0.013	0.036	32.1 (8.4)	28.7 (12.1)	0.225
Women - Column %	-			-	31.1%	62.3%	0.0%	0.009	0.617	30.0%	26.7%	0.803
Men - Column %	-			-	68.9%	37.5%	100.0%			70.0%	73.3%	
White - Column %										78.0%	40.0%	
URM - Column %	-	-	-	-	-	-	-	-	-	14.0%	6.7%	<0.001
Other CALD - Column %										8.0%	53.3%	
Non-White - Column %	-	-	-	-	-	-	-	-	-	22.0%	60.0%	0.005
BDS or Both BDS & DDS/DMD - Column %	10.8%	10.5%	10.9%	0.968	2.2%	12.5%	41.7%	<0.001	<0.001	0.0%	46.7%	<0.001
Master's Degree ≥1 - Column %	72.3%	78.9%	69.6%	0.442	64.4%	86.5%	91.7%	0.102	0.034	72.0%	73.3%	0.919
2nd Doctorate (PhD, MD, JD) - Column %	41.5%	15.8%	52.2%	0.007	44.4%	12.5%	50.0%	0.193	0.476	36.0%	60.0%	**0.098**
Advanced Education (Specialty) - Column %	70.8%	63.2%	73.9%	0.386	62.2%	100%	83.3%	**0.055**	0.023	66.0%	86.7%	0.123
ADA Specialty Boarded - Column %	47.7%	47.4%	47.8%	0.973	40.0%	75.0%	58.3%	0.135	**0.063**	44.0%	60.0%	0.277

Abbreviations: CALD, cultural and linguistical diversity; IDT, international dental training; URM, underrepresented minority.

P<.05 P<.10.

deans, whether man or women, generally are similar. One area of distinction is that more men hold second doctoral degrees. Nearly one-third of the deans are general dentists (**Fig. 4**A), with periodontics and prosthodontics as the highest represented advanced specialty training for the total (see **Fig. 4**A) and among men (**Fig. 4**B). Among the women with the specialties of dental public health, oral pathology, and oral medicine are the most frequent (see **Fig. 4**B).

For school characteristics by gender (**Table 2**), no distributions reach statistically significant difference. The largest difference appears for National Institutes of Health/NIDCR funding where men are more represented at the top 10 and 20 ranking

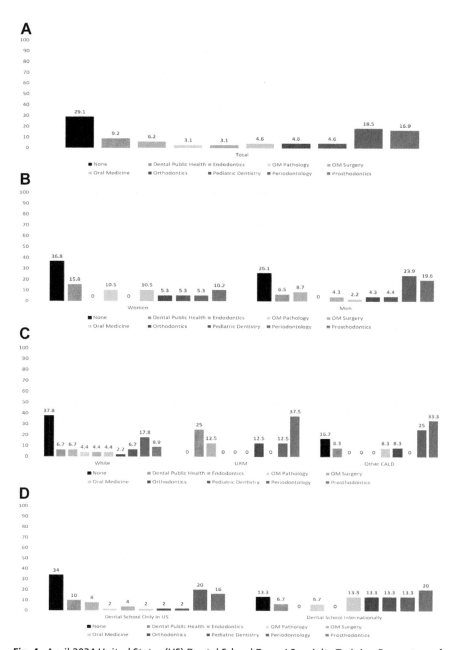

Fig. 4. April 2024 United States (US) Dental School Deans' Specialty Training Percentages for Permanent Deans at US Commission on Dental Accreditation (CODA)-recognized Dental School: (*A*) For Total, (*B*). By Women and Men, (*C*) By Cultural and Linguistic Diversity, and (*D*) By having US only or with International Dental Training.

Table 2
United States dental school characteristics of the April 2024 cohort of permanently named deans at Commission on Dental Accerediton-recognized United States dental schools by gender, cultural and linguistical diversity, and dental degree location

Characteristic	Total	Gender			Cultural and Linguistical Diversity				Non-White	Dental Degree Location		
		Women	Men	P-Value	White	URM	Other CALD	P-Value	P-Value	US Only	International (IDT)	P-Value
Total	65	19	46	-	45	8	12	-	-	50	15	-
(Row %)		(29.2%)	(70.8%)		(69.2%)	(12.3%)	(18.5%)			(78.6%)	(23.1%)	
Central ADEA Region	24.6%	31.6%	21.7%	0.677	26.7%	50.0%	0.0%	0.084	0.513	22.0%	33.3%	0.744
Northeast ADEA Region	21.5%	15.8%	23.9%		24.4%	0.0%	25.0%			24.0%	13.3%	
South ADEA Region	32.3%	36.8%	30.4%		26.7%	50.0%	41.7%			32.0%	33.3%	
West ADEA Region	21.5%	15.8%	23.9%		22.2%	0.0%	33.3%			22.0%	20.0%	
Public	53.8%	47.4%	56.5%	0.501	55.6%	50.0%	50.0%	0.918	0.678	50.0%	66.7%	0.256
Private & Private/State-Related	46.2%	52.6%	43.5%		44.4%	50.0%	50.0%			50.0%	33.3%	
Dean Trained at School	27.7%	36.8%	23.9%	0.289	26.7%	50.0%	16.7%	0.254	0.782	32.0%	13.3%	0.156
State has ≥3 Dental Schools	60.0%	52.6%	63.0%	0.436	57.8%	75.0%	58.3%	0.652	0.582	66.0%	40.0%	0.071
International Degree Program	53.8%	63.2%	50.0%	0.333	51.1%	62.5%	58.3%	0.789	0.507	54.0%	53.3%	0.964
NIH/NIDCR Top 10	15.4%	5.3%	19.6%	0.146	17.8%	12.5%	8.3%	0.702	0.422	16.0%	13.3%	0.802
NIH/NIDCR Top 20	27.7%	15.8%	32.6%	0.168	26.7%	25.0%	33.3%	0.885	0.782	26.0%	33.3%	0.578
NIH/NIDCR Ranked	67.7%	68.4%	67.4%	0.936	64.4%	87.5%	66.7%	0.436	0.401	64.0%	80.0%	0.245

CALD = Cultural and Linguistical Diversity   URM = Underrepresented Minority   IDT = International Dental Training

P<0.1

schools, whereas representation was similar for women and men considering all ranked schools.

Cultural and linguistical diversity
The majority group is White, albeit that the non-White group reaches 30.8% of the deans (see **Table 1**). Among the CALD categories, several differences emerge. The "Other CALD" group on average graduated around a decade more recently have a shorter time between graduation and appointment than "White" and "URM" deans, and are the most represented among deans with a BDS. All deans in the "Other CALD" category are men, while most deans in the URM category are women. Non-White deans are more likely than White deans to have a master's degree and advanced specialty training. All URM deans have specialty training, with high representation in Dental Public Health and Prosthodontics (**Fig. 4**C). None of the URM or other CALD deans have training in OM Pathology, OM Surgery, or Pediatric Dentistry, which are not strongly represented among the White deans. Non-White deans are more likely than White deans to have specialty training and well over half of the non-White deans are specialty boarded, whereas White deans are less than half.

In the consideration of school characteristics for CALD categories (see **Table 2**), no distributions statistically significantly differed; nevertheless, geographic distribution is notable. White deans appear evenly distributed across the ADEA regions. URM deans were evenly split between the Central or South regions, while no "Other CALD" deans were in the Central region and their highest representation was in the South.

International dental training
Among this 2024 dean cohort, almost a quarter had IDT (see **Table 1**). While representation of women is similar between the IDT and US-only dental school training (USDT) groups, a notable difference is in CALD diversity, as most of the IDT deans are non-White, whereas most of the USDT deans are White. Almost half of the IDT deans hold BDS degrees, a degree obviously absent among USDT deans. While similar rates of advanced education training and second doctorates exist, certification by ADA-recognized specialty boards is seen more often among IDT deans, although not reaching statistical difference. The deans with USDT are more likely to be general dentists

(**Fig. 4**D). No IDT deans have training in Endodontics or Oral and Maxillofacial Surgery. While distribution of deans by the 2 sets of training history for most institutional characteristics are similar (see **Table 2**), a suggestion of a different of rate of placement of IDT in states with multiple dental schools is seen with IDT less likely to be in such a location.

DISCUSSION
A Measure of Diversity and Inclusivity

One measure of progress on diversifying and inclusion for leadership is the yardstick of the "30% Solution".[76] The concept of the "30% solution" is that to achieve change, a critical mass is needed, estimated at over 30%, and cannot be achieved by just hiring 1 individual with a particular trait.[76] Promoted in 1995 at the Beijing Fourth United Nations Conference on the Status of Women, the "30% solution" provides direction to leadership equilibrium in the representation of those traditionally underrepresented.[76] Women in the dental workforce broke the "30% solution" threshold in 2017, while non-White individuals did in 2021.[2] Deans appear to be at the cusp of that measure now for both women and non-Whites.

Progress Shown with The April 2024 Dean Cohort

A rise in the number of women deans in dental schools is noted. Women as dental school deans increased almost 15-fold from 1985 to 1986 (1.8%)[77] to the April 2024 data (29.2%). Although still underrepresented, especially as compared to women's representation in the general population and among dental students, this increase is promising and indicates that women are and will become more involved in leadership. A rising trend in women professors, assistant deans, and program chairs in dental academic settings have been reported,[44] with the anticipation that women will continue to progress up through the academic ladders.[77,78]

Integration of wider perspectives, getting dentistry beyond leaders who are "super achievers" appears to be happening. Women are appearing more acceptable as deans for their range on attributes becoming like the men's range. Dentistry appears to be floundering regarding the support of individuals of URM background, in that URM proportions appear stagnant, particularly for Blacks, in the workforce, as well as for being deans (See articles 1[79] and 6[80] in this Issue). Attention must be made to the decline in non-Hispanic Whites being attributable to increases in the other CALD category, rather than in URM and a reflection on continued need for improvement on inclusivity success (See articles 6[80] and 10[81] in this issue).

The presence of IDT dentists in leadership positions can help to address and promote inclusivity and diversity in dental curricula and institutional policies. Their employment aligns with global declarations and initiatives aimed at transforming dental education to meet new societal challenges. For instance, a group of senior scientists meet in 2017 and created "the La Cascada Declaration" emphasizing the need for universal dental education reform in response to global health crises and the importance of inclusivity and equity in health education.[29] Similarly, Townsend and colleagues[82] highlight the evolving demands on dental education leadership, governance, and management, underscoring the importance of adapting to societal changes and fostering a diverse educational environment.

Evaluating This Assessment

This assessment has strengths including that it provides a comprehensive measure of the April 2024 cohort of permanently named deans at CODA-recognized US dental schools. By examining the characteristics of deans through an inclusive lens, it highlights progress in diversity and representation, offering valuable insights into the evolving landscape of dental school leadership. Its holistic approach considers various aspects of diversity, including gender, cultural and linguistic backgrounds, and IDT, providing a multi-dimensional view of inclusivity. The use of publicly available data ensures transparency and replicability. Additionally, by establishing a detailed assessment of the current cohort, this study sets a benchmark for future research on diversity and inclusion in dental school leadership.

Limits of this assessment include overarchingly the fluidity of dental schools and their leadership. Changes in details pertaining to leadership may happen more quickly than updates on websites. Proposed new schools add to the uncertainty of trends. The small numbers of deans in diverse categories impacts statistical testing in general as well restricts the ability to consider intersectionality of attributes. A significant limitation in assessing inclusive environments is that the characteristics measured are proxies for critical variables that are not readily available. Questions about how to measure these traits and whether they are teachable remain ongoing challenges for dentistry and dental education. Furthermore, the reliance on publicly available information may not capture all relevant details. The lack of standardized reporting of information about their deans across institutions also affects data consistency and comparability.

Future Directions Range Across Community, Individuals, and Institutions

Anticipated national population demographic changes, particularly the impact of IDT dentists and dental school leadership, warrant consideration. The Congressional Budget Office projects that starting in 2040, the US population growth will rely on immigration.[83] This demographic shift element adds another dimension to dental workforce development that reflects the country's diversity.

Collecting and reporting the data on the representation of women and other diversity measures in dental leadership, as recommended by the National Academies of Science[46] is important for transparency. **Figs. 1** and **2** in this article illustrate the data gaps and precision problems. Understanding and addressing the challenges of measuring access, presence, and engagement in inclusion efforts will mitigate future issues.

As top executives, deans guide the institution's mission, vision, and values,[84] ensuring high-quality teaching, service, and research.[85] Other health professions have demonstrated the value of diverse leadership, which can enhance patient care, research, and financial management[84,86] and is expanded upon in the interprofessional inclusivity articles[87] in this issue.

Leadership models are dynamic, with a recent focus on inclusion. Inclusive leadership, defined by actions that invite and appreciate others' contributions, creates psychologic safe environments characterized by openness, availability, and accessibility.[88] Key attributes of inclusive leadership include authenticity, collaboration, commitment to diversity, and support for followers.[89] These leaders positively impact students, faculty, and staff, by fostering uniqueness, belonging, creativity and psychologic safety.[89,90]

The environment is shifting from the solo-practitioner needs to multi-practitioner collaboration. An inclusive environment supports diverse faculty recruitment and retention, promoting a culturally diverse workplace.[91] Inclusivity is critical for providing role models and mentors, inspiring faculty members to advance professionally.[92] (See Chapter 10[81]) Expectations for deans to be experts in all areas of clinic, teaching, service, research, innovation, and business are unrealistic. Recently published works, such as the 75th Anniversary Special Issues of the *Journal of Dental Education*[93] and the White Papers Series by the *World Economic Forum*[94,95] are examples of guidance on these shifts.

Leadership Training

As nearly a third of the April 2024 dean cohorts are general dentists, another aspect meeting the "30% Solution[76]", reliance cannot be placed on leadership training occurring at the advanced specialty training level. Other routes for leadership training should be considered, perhaps along the lines of Management of Business Administration, experiences in organized dentistry, or dental specific programs mentioned earlier in the introduction section on women. The preparation of leadership should include the roles of mentorship from perspectives of deans as mentees and mentors, as well as role models benefits the individuals and the institutions (See the articles on mentorship[81] and language[93] in this issue).

Perhaps more attention to leadership training should occur in dental schools. Teaching and applying diversity, equality, and inclusion (DEI) and leadership principles are evolving at the dental student level. The American Student Dental Association as a national dental student-run organization[96] has multiple DEI initiatives, including a "How to Guide: Diversity & Inclusion Workshops".[97] The University of North Carolina dental school has shared an experience with student-focused leadership development of the DEI environment as a model.[98]

Future Overview

Integration into broader aspects of success for inclusive environments in academic dentistry is essential. The performance and impact of deans need measurement of success on the institutions, patients, students, staff faculty, and other leadership, in addition to the general population and interprofessional collaboration. Additionally, the development of standardized metrics is important for assessing inclusivity and diversity, mentorship and leadership training programs, and sustainability of improvements in representation and inclusivity across all levels of dental education and practice.

CLINICS CARE POINTS

- Dental education and practice are increasing expectations for inclusive leadership.
- Historic milestones like the first female and minority dental school deans highlight progress but do not guarantee rapid or complete integration. Ongoing efforts are needed to continue advancing inclusivity.
- The "30% Solution" is a useful benchmark for achieving meaningful representation of women and non-White individuals in leadership roles. While progress has been made in the workforce, this level of representation is still being pursued among dental school deans.
- Awareness of demographic changes in the US population helps to understand and anticipate changes in patient populations and the dental workforce. The demographics of first-year dental students reflect broader societal shifts and are important for planning future educational and leadership initiatives.
- Despite progress, women and historically underrepresented minorities still face challenges in attaining leadership positions in dental education. Continuous efforts are needed to address these disparities.
- The current landscape of dental school leadership includes progress on a mix of genders, ethnic backgrounds, and international training, reflecting an evolving but still incomplete picture of inclusivity.

ACKNOWLEDGMENTS

The authors would like to recognize and thank 2 individuals: Nawal F Dairi, dental student at the University of Pennsylvania School of Dental Medicine and former research volunteer at the University of Illinois Chicago College of Dentistry for her fundamental contributions to initial work, and Dr Evelina Kratunova, Clinical Associate Professor at the University of Illinois Chicago College of Dentistry, who with international dental training, provided valuable insight across the article.

DISCLOSURE

The authors disclose no commercial or financial conflicts of interest or any funding resources for this Dental Clinics article.

REFERENCES

1. United States census bureau. Available at: www.census.gov. Accessed May 13, 2024.
2. American Dental Association Health Policy Institute. U.S. Dentist demographics dashboard. Available at: https://www.ada.org/resources/research/health-policy-institute/us-dentist-demographics. Accessed May 13, 2024.
3. American Dental Association Health Policy Institute. Trends in U.S. Dental schools. Available at: https://www.ada.org/-/media/project/ada-organization/ada/ada-org/files/resources/research/hpi/hpigraphic_0821_1.pdf?rev=99a898d70dac4ce4a6de52f4b29bac4e&hash=A6433BBBBF716E78C01354BC739CC6E8. Accessed May 28, 2024.
4. American Dental Association Health Policy Institute. Racial and ethnic mix of dental students in the U.S. Available at: https://www.ada.org/-/media/project/ada-organization/ada/ada-org/files/resources/research/hpi/HPIgraphic_0421_2.pdf?la=en#:~:text=Nearly%20one%2Dquarter%20of%20dental,6%25%20of%20the%20U.S.%20population.&text=Source%3A%20ADA%20Health%20Policy%20Institute%20analysis%20of%20data,the%20American%20Dental%20Education%20Association. Accessed May 28, 2024.
5. Valachovic RW, Weaver RG, Haden NK, et al. A profile of dental school deans. J Dent Educ 2000;64(6):433-9.
6. Haden NK, Ditmyer MM, Rodriguez T, et al. A profile of dental school deans, 2014. J Dent Educ 2015;79(10):1243-50.
7. Bompolaki D, Pokala SV, Koka S. Gender diversity and senior leadership in academic dentistry: female representation at the dean position in the United States. J Dent Educ 2022;86(4):401-5.
8. Brown LJ, Wagner KS, Johns B. Racial/ethnic variations of practicing dentists. J Am Dent Assoc 2000;131(12):1750-4.
9. Loevy HT, Kowitz AA. Women dentists, Hobbs and after. J Hist Dent 2002;50(3):123-30.
10. Dummett CO. A historical perspective of thirteen unheralded contributors to medicodental progress. J Natl Med Assoc 1989;81(3):307-20.
11. Dummett CO. Dentistry's beginnings among blacks in the United States. J Natl Med Assoc 1974;66(4):321-7.
12. Agbor-Taylor P. 2013, november 22). Ida Gray Nelson Rollins (1867-1953. Available at: https://www.blackpast.org/african-american-history/rollins-ida-gray-nelson-1867-1953/. Accessed May 8, 2024.

13. Chiu GK, Davies WI. The historical development of dentistry in Hong Kong. Hong Kong Med J 1998;4(1):73–6.
14. University of Michigan School of Dentistry Sindecuse Museum. Faith Sai So Leong (1884-1929). Available at: https://www.sindecusemuseum.org/faith-sai-so-leong. Accessed June 4, 2024.
15. Mikkelsen E. 2007, january 17). Arnold Bennett Donowa (1896-1964. Available at: https://www.blackpast.org/african-american-history/donowa-arnold-bennett-1896-196/. Accessed May 8, 2024.
16. Dental international student program at Tufts university school of dental medicine. Available at: https://programs.adea.org/CAAPID/programs/tufts-university-school-of-dental-medicine. Accessed June 4, 2024.
17. Blue Spruce G, Durrett D. Searching for My Destiny (American Indian Lives). Lincoln, NE: Bison Books University of Nebraska Press; 2012. p. 336.
18. Reidar F. Sognnaes, LDS, PhD, DMD: the thirty-fourth president of IADR, 1957-58. J Dent Res 1984;63:11.
19. Reidar fouske sognnaes. Wikipedia. Available at: https://en.wikipedia.org/wiki/Reidar_Fauske_Sognnaes#cite_note-1. Accessed May 16, 2024.
20. Jeanne C., Sinkford In: Price S.S., Sinkford J.C., Woolfolk M.P.. Undaunted Trailblazers: Minority Women Leaders for Oral Health. American Dental Education Association; Washington, DC, 2021. 181-187.
21. University of Michigan School of Dentistry Sindecuse Museum. Meet an American Indian dentist, advocate, and role model: jessica rickert. 2021. Available at: https://www.sindecusemuseum.org/blog/jessica-rickert-dds. Accessed March 19, 2024.
22. Wikipedia. University of Puerto Rico school of dental medicine. Available at: https://en.wikipedia.org/wiki/University_of_Puerto_Rico_School_of_Dental_Medicine. Accessed May 9, 2024.
23. Mary Lynne Capilouto. Personal Communication. (Accessed 27 June 2024).
24. University of California Los Angeles. profile: No-Hee Park, D.M.D., Ph.D. Available at: https://dentistry.ucla.edu/profile/park-no-hee. Accessed May 17, 2024.
25. Bailit HL, Formicola AJ, Herbert KD, et al. The origins and design of the Dental Pipeline program. J Dent Educ 2005;69(2):232–8.
26. University of Puerto Rico School of Dental Medicine. Personal Contact via estudianesdental.rcm@upr.edu. (Accessed 17 June 2024).
27. Sahingur SE. Dr. Marjorie K. Jeffcoat - a renaissance woman in oral health sciences and education. Oral Dis 2023;29(Suppl 1):890–2.
28. Wikipedia. Rena D'Souza. Available at: https://en.wikipedia.org/wiki/Rena_D%27Souza. Accessed June 20, 2024.
29. Cohen LC, Dahlen G, Escobar A, et al. Dentistry in crisis: time to change. La Cascada Declaration. Aust Dent J 2017;62(3):258–60.
30. Kalkwarf KL. Creating multicultural dental schools and the responsibility of leadership. J Dent Educ 1995;59(12):1107–10.
31. Prasad JL, Rojek MK, Gordon SC, et al. Sex and gender health educational tenets: an essential paradigm for inclusivity in dentistry – this issue of DCNA
32. Rivera CJ, Jimenez BA, Baker JN, et al. A culturally and linguistically responsive framework for improving academic and postsecondary outcomes of students with moderate or severe intellectual disability. PDERS 2016;35(2):23–48.
33. Ginsburgh VA, Weber S. Chapter 19. Culture, linguistic diversity, and economics. In: Ginsburg VA, Throsby D, editors. Handbook of the economics of art and culture, 2. Elsevier BV; 2024. p. 507–43.

34. Loevy HT, Kowitz AA. Dental education for women dentists in the United States: the beginnings. Quintessence Int 1999;30(8):563–9.
35. Neidle EA. President's address. J Dent Educ 1986;50(7):380–2.
36. Sinkford JC, Valachovic RW, Harrison S. Advancement of women in dental education: trends and strategies. J Dent Educ 2003;67(1):79–83.
37. ADA HPI 2021 infographic. Available at: https://www.ada.org/-/media/project/ada-organization/ada/ada-org/files/resources/research/hpi/hpigraphic_0821_1.pdf?rev=99a898d70dac4ce4a6de52f4b29bac4e&hash=A6433BBBBF716E78C01354BC739CC6E8. Accessed May 17, 2024.
38. Gies WJ. Dental education in the United States and Canada bulletin number nineteen (the gies report). The Carnegie Foundation for the Advancement of Teaching; 1926. p. 40.
39. Wikipedia. Eugenia L. Mobley. Available at: https://en.wikipedia.org/wiki/Eugenia_L._Mobley#cite_note-:1-11. Accessed June 28, 2024.
40. Clevenger S. OHSU school of dentistry: 114 Years and growing. CAEMENTUM: OHSU school of dentistry winter. 2013. Available at: https://www.ohsu.edu/sites/default/files/2019-07/caementum_winter13_FINAL_pages_0.pdf. Accessed June 28, 2024.
41. University hospital New Jersey. Cecile A. Feldman, DMD, MBA. Available at: https://www.uhnj.org/about-us/board-of-directors/cecile-a-feldman-dmd-mba/. Accessed July 1, 2024.
42. A conversation with martha somerman. University of Washington. Available at: https://www.washington.edu/news/2007/02/22/a-conversation-with-martha-somerman-dean-of-the-school-of-dentistry/. Accessed June 21, 2024.
43. AEGIS dental network, women advancing dentistry. 2009. Available at: https://www.aegisdentalnetwork.com/special-issues/2009/12/women-advancing-dentistry. Accessed May 17, 2024.
44. University of Florida. Teresa A dolan, Prof emeritus & dean emeritus. Available at: https://dental.ufl.edu/profile/dolan-teresa/. Accessed July 1, 2024.
45. Yuan JC, Lee DJ, Kongkiatkamon S, et al. Gender trends in dental leadership and academics: a twenty-two-year observation. J Dent Educ 2010;74(4):372–80.
46. Kim A, Karra N, Song C, et al. Gender trends in dentistry: dental faculty and academic leadership. J Dent Educ 2024;88(1):23–9.
47. Ioannidou E, D'Souza RN, Macdougall MJ. Gender equity in dental academics: gains and unmet challenges. J Dent Res 2014;93(1):5–7.
48. National Academies of Sciences, Engineering, and Medicine. Promising practices for addressing the underrepresentation of women in science, engineering, and medicine: opening doors. Washington, DC: The National Academies Press; 2020.
49. Whelton H, Wardman MJ. The landscape for women leaders in dental education, research, and practice. J Dent Educ 2015;79(5 Suppl):S7–12.
50. Cohen DW. The development and progress of the executive leadership in academic medicine program for women (ELAM), 1993-98. J Dent Educ 1999;63(3):238–9.
51. Dannels SA, McLaughlin JM, Gleason KA, et al. Dental school deans' perceptions of the organizational culture and impact of the ELAM program on the culture and advancement of women faculty. J Dent Educ 2009;73(6):676–88.
52. Haden NK, Ditmyer MM, Mobley C, et al. Leadership development in dental education: report on the ADEA leadership Institute, 2000-14. J Dent Educ 2016; 80(4):478–87.

53. Garcia MN, Andrews EA, White CC, et al. Advancing women, parity, and gender equity. J Dent Educ 2022;86(9):1182–90.
54. Weinstein GJ, Haden NK, Stewart DCL, et al. A profile of dental school deans, 2021. J Dent Educ 2022;86(10):1304–16.
55. Perspectives of change: dolores mercedes Franklin, DMD, class of 1974 (first african American woman to graduate from HSDM). Available at: https://perspectivesofchange.hms.harvard.edu/node/115. Accessed May 9, 2024.
56. The HBCU Career Center. Top HBCU dental schools for aspiring dentists and dental hygienists. Available at: https://www.thehbcucareercenter.com/blog/top-hbcu-dental-schools-for-aspiring-dentists-and-dental-hygienists. Accessed May 8, 2024.
57. Ferris State University, Russell A. Dixon - january 2017 – question of the month – jim crow museum. Available at: https://jimcrowmuseum.ferris.edu/question/2017/January.htm. Accessed May 8, 2024.
58. Dummett CO. National Museum of Dentistry exhibition: the future is now! African Americans in dentistry. J Natl Med Assoc 2003;95(9):879–83.
59. Charles Goodall lee. Available at: https://en.wikipedia.org/wiki/Charles_Goodall_Lee. Accessed May 13, 2024.
60. Laden BV. Hispanic-serving institutions: what are they? Where are they? Community College. J Res Pract 2004;28:181–98.
61. National Center for Educational Statistics. Table 312.40. Enrollment and degrees conferred in degree-granting Hispanic-serving institutions, by institution level and control, percentage Hispanic, degree level, and other selected characteristics: fall 2021 and academic year 2020-21. Available at: https://nces.ed.gov/programs/digest/d22/tables/dt22_312.40.asp. Accessed May 10, 2024.
62. American Indian Higher Education Consortium. Tribal Colleges & Universities. Available at: https://www.aihec.org/tribal-colleges-universities/. Accessed May 9, 2024.
63. Atchison KA, Thind A, Carreon DC, et al. Comparison of extramural clinical rotation days: did the Pipeline program make a difference? J Dent Educ 2011;75(1):52–61.
64. Pew Research Center. A changing World: global views on diversity, gender equality, family life and the importance of religion. Available at: www.pewresearch.org. Accessed May 28, 2024.
65. Hojat M, DeSantis J, Shannon SC, et al. Empathy as related to gender, age, race and ethnicity, academic background and career interest: a nationwide study of osteopathic medical students in the United States. Med Educ 2020;54(6):571–81.
66. Batra S, Orban J, Zhang H, et al. Analysis of social mission commitment at dental, medical, and nursing schools in the US. JAMA Netw Open 2022;5(5):e2210900.
67. Till MJ, Posnick WR, Walker JD. Toward solving the manpower shortage in dental education. A look at recruitment. J Am Coll Dent 1975;42(4):230–40.
68. Haden NK, Weaver RG, Valachovic RW. Meeting the demand for future dental school faculty: trends, challenges, and responses. J Dent Educ 2002;66(9):1102–13.
69. Flores-Mir C. Dental faculty shortage in the United States and Canada: are there solutions? J Can Dent Assoc 2006;72(8):725–6.
70. Knechtel ME. A proposal to alleviate faculty shortages in dental schools. J Can Dent Assoc 2007;73(9):815–7.
71. Bazargan N, Chi DL, Milgrom P. Exploring the potential for foreign-trained dentists to address workforce shortages and improve access to dental care for

vulnerable populations in the United States: a case study from Washington State. BMC Health Serv Res 2010;10:336.

72. Keels MA, Kaste LM, Weintraub JA, et al. A national survey of women dentists. J Am Dent Assoc 1991;122(12):31–3, 36–7,40-33.

73. Allareddy V, Elangovan S, Nalliah RP, et al. Pathways for foreign-trained dentists to pursue careers in the United States. J Dent Educ 2014;78(11):1489–96.

74. ADEA centralized application for advanced placement for international dentists. Available at: https://www.adea.org/adeacaapid/. Accessed May 22, 2024.

75. ADEA CAAPID® programs. Available at: https://programs.adea.org/CAAPID/programs. Accessed May 22, 2024.

76. Tarr-Whelan L. Women lead the way: your guide to stepping up to leadership and changing the World. San Francisco, CA: Berrett-Koehlers Publishers, Inc.; 2009.

77. Reed MJ, Corry AM, Liu YW. The role of women in dental education: monitoring the pipeline to leadership. J Dent Educ 2012;76(11):1427–36.

78. Li J, de Souza R, Esfandiari S, et al. Have women broken the glass ceiling in North American dental leadership? Adv Dent Res 2019;30(3):78–84.

79. Halpern LR, Kaste LM, Southerland JH. The I in DEI: Conveying inclusion, belonging and equity. – This issue of DCNA.

80. Fleming E, Perez HL. Inclusion in Dentistry – This issue of DCNA.

81. Evolution of Mentoring in Fostering Inclusion, led by Leslie R. Halpern, in this DCNA issue.

82. Townsend G, Thomas R, Skinner V, et al. Leadership, governance and management in dental education - new societal challenges. Eur J Dent Educ 2008; 12(Suppl 1):131–48.

83. Congressional Budget Office. The demographic outlook: 2024 to 2054. 2024. Available at: https://www.cbo.gov/publication/59697. Accessed May 28, 2024.

84. Jacobson CE, Beeler WH, Griffith KA, et al. Common pathways to Dean of Medicine at U.S. medical schools. PLoS One 2021;16(3):e0249078.

85. Trainor R. What the head of a university expects from the leadership of a dental school. J Dent 2019;87:62–5.

86. Beeler WH, Cortina LM, Jagsi R. Diving beneath the surface: addressing gender inequities among clinical investigators. J Clin Invest 2019;129(9):3468–71.

87. Models for Inclusion in DEIB from Other Health Professions led by Janet Southerland – this issue of DCNA.

88. Nembhard IM, Edmondson AC. Making it safe: the effects of leader inclusiveness and professional status on psychological safety and improvement efforts in health care teams. J Organiz Behav 2006;27(7):941–66.

89. Fagan HAS, Wells B, Guenther S, et al. The path to inclusion: a literature review of attributes and impacts of inclusive leaders. J Leadership Educ 2022;21(1): 88–113.

90. Fu Q, Cherian J, Ahmad N, et al. An inclusive leadership framework to foster employee creativity in the healthcare sector: the role of psychological safety and polychronicity. Int J Environ Res Publ Health 2022;19(8):4519.

91. Kamran SC, Winkfield KM, Reede JY, et al. Intersectional analysis of U.S. Medical faculty diversity over four decades. N Engl J Med 2022;386(14):1363–71.

92. Feldman CA. Attaining and sustaining leadership for U.S. women in dentistry. J Dent Educ 2015;79(5 Suppl):S13–7.

93. Sinkford JC, Smith SG. Introduction to this special issue. J Dent Educ 2022;86(9): 1051–4.

94. White papers: the economic rationale for a global commitment to invest in oral health. 2024. Available at: https://www.weforum.org/publications/the-economic-

rationale-for-a-global-commitment-to-invest-in-oral-health/. Accessed May 29, 2024.

95. Haley CM, Doubleday AF. Inclusive Language to Support Equity and Belonging in Dentistry, in this DCNA issue.

96. American student dental association. Available at: https://www.asdanet.org/about-asda. Accessed June 4, 2024.

97. American Student Dental Association. How-to guide: diversity & inclusion workshops. Available at: https://www.asdanet.org/docs/publications/how-to-guides/dei-education-how-to-guide_final.pdf. Accessed May 28, 2024.

98. Kornegay EC, Hayon E, Gisler S, et al. Preparing learners to ACT as change agents: early implementation of leadership curricula in dental education. J Dent Educ 2023;87(9):1257–70.

Ageism and Ableism in Individuals Aging with Intellectual and Developmental Disabilities

Christine Wieseler, PhD[a], Elisa M. Chávez, DDS[b],
Janet A. Yellowitz, DMD, MPH[c],*

KEYWORDS

• Ableism • Ageism • Inclusivity • Aging • Bioethics • Dentistry • Inclusion

KEY POINTS

• Individuals with Intellectual and Developmental Disabilities (IDD) experience accelerated aging.
• Ageism and Ableism are essential barriers to inclusivity for individuals with IDD.
• Individuals who have long dealt with ableism often encounter biases and barriers to oral health care as a result of ageism as they experience increasing dependency as a result of age prevalent diseases.
• New challenges to independence may require managing transitions in care with implications for oral disease prevention and maintaining oral health over a lifetime.

INTRODUCTION

This article will define and discuss the significance of ableism and ageism for those aging with Intellectual and Developmental Disabilities (IDD) seeking oral health care. We will discuss accelerated aging in individuals with IDD and the consequences for oral health. Until the latter part of the 20th century, most individuals with IDD experienced markedly shortened life expectancies, particularly in institutional residences.[1] Improvements in medical care have led to longer lifespans for people with disabilities. As adults aging with IDD live longer and with greater independence, providers face unique assessment and treatment challenges. Health care providers can play a pivotal

^a Department of Philosophy, Santa Clara University, 500 EL Camino Real, Santa Clara, CA 95053, USA; ^b Diagnostic Sciences, Pacific Center for Equity in Oral Health Care, University of the Pacific, Arthur A. Dugoni School of Dentistry, 155 5th Street, 4th Floor, San Francisco, CA 94103, USA; ^c Geriatric Dentistry, University of Maryland School of Dentistry, 650 West Baltimore Street #3211, Baltimore, MD 21201, USA
* Corresponding author.
E-mail address: Jyellowitz@umaryland.edu

Dent Clin N Am 69 (2025) 103–114
https://doi.org/10.1016/j.cden.2024.08.005
0011-8532/25/© 2024 Elsevier Inc. All rights reserved, including those for text and data mining, AI training, and similar technologies.
dental.theclinics.com

role in promoting, managing, and delivering care that supports a high quality of life for older adults with IDD.[1] Since oral health plays an important role in overall health and wellbeing, it is essential to address oral health concerns for aging individuals with IDD, who have an increased likelihood of developing chronic diseases.

Bioethicist Erik Parens advocates *binocular thinking* about disability, meaning considering the effects of the biomedical conditions of individuals in tandem with ways that assumptions about disability and social practices create or reduce opportunities for people with disabilities.[2] Sometimes medical interventions can be the best way to promote the flourishing of people with disabilities, but, in many cases, changes to the social/physical environment are the priority. Indeed, both may be necessary. Even though we can make a conceptual distinction, the 2 aspects of binocular thinking about disability influence each other. For example, some of the diseases that aging people with IDD experience may result in a new or increased level of dependency. Parents of, and many baby boomers with IDD had few publicly funded family and community services, with institutional care and services the norm. Due to disability activism, legislation, and changes to social norms over the past several decades, there is greater access, choice, and control over services, which allows some individuals with IDD to gain and retain their independence. Increased dependency in older age can be particularly challenging for adults who may have struggled with ablest stereotypes to gain or maintain their independence over a lifetime. New challenges to independence may require managing transitions in care with implications for oral disease prevention and maintaining oral health over a lifetime. Throughout this article, we will employ binocular thinking to examine biomedical and structural factors that impact oral health for people with IDD.

The Centers for Disease Control and Prevention reports that about 27% of the population in the United States has some kind of impairment, with cognitive (12.8%) and mobility impairments (12.1%) being the most common.[3] According to the US Census Bureau, the number of people 65 and over "reached 55.8 million or 16.8% of the population of the United States in 2020".[4] Approximately 35% of Americans 65 and older are disabled, and about 41% of disabled people are 65 and older.[5] The number of adults with IDD age 60 years and older is projected to reach an estimated 1.2 million by 2030 when the baby boom generation will be over 65 years of age. National Core Indicators (NCI) data describe the characteristics of older adults with IDD.[6] Data from 2017 to 2018 indicate that those under age 55 are more likely to have diagnoses of autism spectrum disorder or cerebral palsy compared with older cohorts. The proportion of the sample reported to have Down syndrome (DS) decreased with increasing age, likely given the onset of Alzheimer's disease that is nearly 20 years earlier than the general population, owing to a shorter life expectancy.[6]

The average lifespan for someone with IDD is 66 years old, compared to 77 years old among the general population.[7] Lifespan varies depending on their diagnosis, with the lowest for those with cerebral palsy, whose average life expectancy is 51[7]. People with IDD have experienced an increased life expectancy along with the broader population; however, this increase is lower overall than the general population and often accompanied by accelerated aging.

ACCELERATED AGING IN INDIVIDUALS WITH INTELLECTUAL AND DEVELOPMENTAL DISABILITIES AND CONSEQUENCES FOR ORAL HEALTH

Accelerated Aging refers to the early onset of health conditions associated with aging among people with disabilities. Adults with IDD are more likely to develop chronic health conditions at younger ages than other adults because of biological factors related to syndromes and associated developmental disabilities, limited access to adequate health care, and lifestyle and environmental issues. Accelerated aging is the difference between biological and chronologic age. Biological age is often derived from a combination of biomarkers that include but are not limited to: total cholesterol, high-density lipoprotein (HDL), glucose, body mass index (BMI) and others that represent the physiologic effects of "wear and tear" usually associated with chronologic aging.[8] Differences in mortality across race and ethnicity among people with IDD follow the same trends as in the general populations.[9] Heart disease is the leading cause of death for all adults 65 and older, with or without IDD.[7] Cancer and diabetes follow for those with mild to moderate IDD but for those with profound IDD, pneumonia and influenza were second and third, with an increased risk of death from choking. There is also an earlier age of onset of and increased risk of death from Alzheimer's disease.[9] Understanding these causes of death is important because these conditions and the medications used to treat them can result in specific risks to oral health.[10]

The most common cause of IDD is DS (or trisomy 21). Persons with DS are inclined to a shorter lifespan. The reason for the unrelenting shorter lifespan in the DS population, compared to many other developmental disability populations, is thought to be due to an accelerated aging process, which is manifested by an increased risk for heart problems, metabolic syndrome, cataracts, hearing loss, osteopenia/osteoporosis, hypothyroidism, and Alzheimer's disease. Moreover, individuals with DS have unique physiologic and physical characteristics, such as muscle hypotonicity, joint hypermobility, and increased tendency for obesity.[11,12]

In one study, individuals with disabilities reported greater rates of hypertension, arthritis, joint pain, and difficulties with vision.[13] For those 65+ years, adults with disabilities reported greater frequency of organ system diseases (diabetes, coronary artery disease and cancer) than those age-matched without disabilities. Health care providers need to be aware of the health needs associated with rapid organ system decline in individuals with IDD. To achieve optimal outcomes, these conditions must be considered when designing treatment plans and planning patient management strategies for patients with IDD in mid or later life. In addition to understanding implications of early onset of chronic diseases, it is necessary to consider how ableism and ageism impact oral health outcomes.

THE INTERSECTION OF ABLEISM AND AGEISM

Aging individuals with IDD will likely have to contend with issues of ageism and ableism as they face the onset of age-associated chronic diseases and conditions. As a result, some seek to avoid being perceived as disabled or old, while others try to hide their disability or refuse to identify as disabled; many aging people resist identifying as old. Both identities carry stigma and the likelihood that others will treat one differently, whether making assumptions about one's capacities, offering unwanted help, or discounting one's value.[5] Individuals who identify as Black, Indigenous, and people of color (BIPOC) and/or LGBTQ+ of all ages with impairments and chronic illnesses may not identify as disabled, as an attempt to avoid additional marginalization or because of a historical lack of inclusivity in their communities and a failure to affirm all aspects of their identity.[14]

Many euphemisms refer to old and disabled people.[5,15,16] The intention of these social and linguistic practices may be kindness, but the unintended effects include erasure of the experiences of those who fall into these categories and continued stigmatization. For example, when a provider denies a person's status as old, the assumption that being old is inherently bad and the concept is not challenged. The same is true when a disabled person is told that providers tell patients that they "don't think of them as disabled." Likewise, the claim that "we are all disabled" ignores the differences between those who are subject to ableism and those who are not. Joel Michael Reynolds contends that "ableism is at the core of ageism" and we "cannot conceptualize ageism without ableism."[17]

The influential model of "successful aging," developed by gerontologists John Rowe and Robert Kahn, serve as a useful example of how ageism and ableism intersect.[18] They "aimed to identify the factors that lead some people to an ideal version of aging marked by mental and physical vitality, as opposed to 'usual aging' which involves some inevitable decline."[5] "Success" requires that one maintain exceptionally high levels of physical and cognitive function, avoid disease and impairment, and is "actively engaged in life."[5] Although these may seem to be useful metrics, this approach has significant limitations. For example, as Lamb[5] characterizes the position of Hailee Gibbons:[19] "successful aging discourse falsely presents being old and being disabled as choices—the result of an individual's lifelong behaviors."[5,19] Not only does this framework fail to account for factors outside of the control of individuals, but it also excludes, by definition, the possibility that disabled people can age successfully.[5] Ageism and ableism are so pervasive within our society that it can be difficult to think critically about the assumptions and practices premised on them. Yet, it is essential that health care providers do so if they are to have any hope of changing these assumptions of inclusivity and create a society that values all *bodyminds*—a term Margaret Price coined to emphasize the intertwined nature of our bodies and minds—rather than only those that are meet the ideal of being young and nondisabled.[20]

Nondisabled and/or young people often assume that being disabled and/or old is a fact or set of facts about an individual that automatically leads to a reduced quality of life however, significant empirical evidence supports that this is not the case. The built environment and the attitudes that inform how it is built and maintained *do* significantly impact quality of life, for better or worse.[21–25]

The Americans with Disabilities Act (ADA) of 1990, along with subsequent updates, was groundbreaking in establishing legal requirements for access and recourse for people with disabilities who face unjust discrimination.[26] To some extent, responsibility for accessibility shifted from disabled individuals to business owners. As monumental as this law was it would be a mistake to believe that it has led to a nation that is perfectly accessible to disabled people. It is still common for health care providers to be insufficiently familiar with its requirements. Furthermore, even when health care facilities comply with the law this does not guarantee that they are fully accessible and welcoming to disabled people. The ADA 1990 provided a good starting point, but it is necessary to attend to the experiences of disabled patients to learn where it falls short.[27]

Consider examples of how some of the needs of disabled and old people are relevant within clinical spaces. Communication is foundational to providing quality care and access to all patients. The awkwardness of not knowing how to engage with disabled people and the stigma around disability and old age compromises good communication. Too often, clinicians are navigating unfamiliar situations and make errors due to their unfamiliarity of best practices. For instance, when patients use American Sign Language or other type of interpreter, it is important for clinicians to talk and make eye contact with the patient rather than with the interpreter. The same is true in instances in which a disabled patient has someone who accompanies them during appointments to provide support, regardless of the form that support takes (eg, assistance with decision making, physical transfers, managing anxiety, speaking on behalf of a person unable to speak). This simple shift can make the difference between a patient feeling ignored or respected in their interactions with clinicians.[28]

Different considerations come to the fore in communication with individuals who develop hearing impairments later in life. "If communication with a late-deafened individual is difficult due to a lack of residual hearing, a health care worker with time pressures may be more likely to presume choices or hurry through the process rather than take the time to ensure that effective communication has occurred."[28] Similarly, older individuals seeking to avoid the stigma of having a disability may engage in what Burke calls "bluffing"—attempting to mask the degree of their hearing impairment.[29] For these reasons, it is important for clinicians to ask patients questions to assess their capabilities and comprehension of the information presented. Providing treatment plans in writing is helpful for most people, but especially those with hearing impairments and/or IDD. When clinic staff know that communication with a patient may take longer than it does with a typical patent, scheduling longer appointments can help to alleviate time pressures.

Beyond the walls of the clinic, disabled and/or old people can face a variety of obstacles to accessing dental care and following the recommendations of clinicians. *Systems analysis* is a method employed within bioethics that asserts the importance of attending to factors outside of an individual's control that constrains the choices available to them. To be inclusive these external factors and the role they play in a patient's ability to access care and to successful outcomes must be considered, this method "can help us to see the difference between when people are 'making bad choices' and when people only 'have bad choices' to choose from."[30] For example, adequate accessible transportation remains out of reach within many communities or can be hit or miss. Anyone who needs a wheelchair lift to ride the bus is familiar with the experiences of encountering buses with broken wheelchair lifts.[28,31] In some places, paratransit is an alternative available to disabled individuals, yet often they are underfunded and unpredictable, which can result in long wait times and late pickups.[28] Arriving late for appointments is a common result, which can frustrate providers and, reflects poorly on patients only to reinforce negative stereotypes about individuals who are disabled or old when in fact the systems to support them have failed or are lacking altogether.

BIOMEDICAL AND STRUCTURAL CHALLENGES INTELLECTUAL AND DEVELOPMENTAL DISABILITIES FACE IN MAINTAINING ORAL HEALTH

Adults with IDD generally see primary health care providers (physicians and dentists) less often compared with the general population, resulting in reduced access to preventive care, screenings, and health inequities between those with IDD and their peers without IDD (**Box 1**). Obtaining and maintenance of good oral health, requires conscientious daily home care and routine professional oral health care. Many older adults with IDD need support to achieve optimal oral health outcomes.[32,33] These adults experience higher rates of obesity and poor nutritional habits, and they often present with more oral health conditions compared with the general population. Numerous studies have found that adults with IDD are more likely to have poor oral hygiene, periodontal disease and untreated dental caries compared with members of the general population.[32,34] Poor oral health is not only due to their limitations to complete good daily oral care, to cooperate during professional dental visits, and medications that affect oral health, but also high rates of poverty. These issues are exacerbated in older adults who have experienced poverty and poor access to dental care throughout their entire lifetime.[34–37] Barriers people with IDD face in accessing dental care include dental practices not accepting them as patients due to financial disincentives (eg, Medicaid's low reimbursement rates) and the scarcity of dental professionals trained

---

Box 1
Reasons individuals with IDD see primary care providers less often than the general population[1,12]

- Limited access to knowledgeable and experienced primary care providers
- Sensory and/or behavioral issues that impact the person's ability to cooperate with examinations and evaluations
- Physical challenges that may limit access to a health care facility
- Decreased ability of individuals with IDD to self-report signs and symptoms of illness
- Individuals with IDD and their caregivers overlooking subtle changes in physical health
- Confusion between conditions associated with IDD and symptoms of an acquired cognitive impairment
- Individuals and/or their caregivers unaware of the need for routine oral health assessments
- Difficulty measuring changes in level of functioning over time
- Diagnostic overshadowing

---

to serve patients with IDD.[38–40] Issues related to informed consent may also present barriers to dental care.[41] Without adequate personal and professional care, individuals with IDD are at greater risk for developing severe oral diseases, as these are progressive when left untreated. Extensive dental caries and periodontal disease result in poor oral health and/or edentulism and the need for removable prostheses, which often are poorly tolerated in those with IDD and those with oral motor function disturbances.[10]

The implications of poor oral health are substantial, with research highlighting the impact poor oral health has on general health, including significant associations with aspiration pneumonia and major chronic diseases such as cardiovascular disease, diabetes, respiratory disease, and stroke.[42–44] Oral health also has an important influence on an individual's psychological and social health. Poor oral health can lead to toothache, associated anxiety, difficulty performing daily activities, impaired social interactions and reduced nutritional intake.[45]

TRANSITIONS IN CARE AND IMPLICATIONS FOR ORAL HEALTH CARE

For many adults with IDD, the transition to adulthood comes with diminished resources for care, including the loss of previously coordinated care.[46] While the Children's Health Insurance Program and the Patient Protection and Affordable Care Act expansion greatly improved access to dental benefits for children, adult oral health care benefits available through Medicaid vary from state to state.[47] While there has been significant expansion of benefits across several states, they are still highly variable and there are no requirements about the kinds of procedures provided.[47] Even when there are benefits available, there may be limited provider participation that restricts access to care. Provider participation is more limited for those in rural areas or individuals who require specialized care, such as those with IDD. For those with the added complexity of accelerated aging, the problem of access to providers and a lack of benefits as adults compounds the problem of access to care. Routine dental services are expressly excluded from Medicare.[47,48] Access to dentistry expressly excludes and is limited to a very few patients who qualify based on medical necessity as defined by Centers for Medicare and Medicaid Services (CMS) for services such as dental examinations and treatment of dental related infection for those preparing for heart valve replacement, organ transplants or treatment for cancers of the head and neck.[48] For those who have experienced financial burdens over a lifetime, few resources are available to offset the loss of dental benefits that may have been available as a child. All the efforts at prevention in childhood can easily be erased in adulthood when access to care is limited,

A lack of coordination exists between service providers for those with IDD and aging services.[46,49] Services aimed at older adults may not appropriately address the needs of those with IDD and those who serve the needs of those with IDD may be ill prepared to meet the needs of those with disabilities associated with aging.[50] For those with IDD who experience diseases and conditions that diminish the ability to preserve what may have been hard-won independence and autonomy in the face of stigma and ableism, it can be difficult to accept the need for a transition in care or the acceptance of help with activities and personal care. Individuals who once lived independently might require assisted living or a skilled nursing level of care due to progressive or debilitating conditions in later life. A lack of coordinated services to navigate these transitions can add to disparities in care and poor outcomes.[46,50]

Limited studies exist about caregivers for older adults with IDD, but it is known that family caregivers age alongside their child, or sibling.[51,52] Care needs often become more complex due to chronic diseases combined with ongoing needs. Aging caregivers may also experience increasing health needs. For caregivers of those with an acquired disability in the general population, there is an estimated period of 4.5 years of caregiving. For those who have children or siblings with IDD, this caregiving can be for most of their lifetime, often with sustained intensity. Some caregivers, referred to as compound or "club sandwich" caregivers provide care for their adult children or siblings with a disability as well as aging parents. These caregivers are more likely to consider placing family members in residential care. Many are primary caregivers with jobs that lack the option of taking a family leave or who must forgo paid employment altogether to care for their family members. The lacking resources of time and money can leave individuals and families too depleted to seek needed oral health care. One study found that sibling caregivers tended to be older, married and with greater incomes when they assumed caregiving duties. They also demonstrated greater engagement with advocacy, future planning, and more positive relationships with the individual than parental or other caregivers.

Dental providers must be prepared to identify and manage the risks to oral health that come from increased dependence for daily oral care and access to dental providers.[53] This preparation requires an understanding of the level of dependence and the day-to-day environment that plays a role in their oral hygiene at home or in a care facility. Likewise, providers must be prepared with preventive strategies to preserve autonomy and oral health at the same time. This can be a challenge for those who are resistant to receiving assistance with oral care, or for those whose caregivers have a limited knowledge or ability to provide adequate daily home care.[10,53] As oral care routines change over a lifetime increasing dependence requires special attention to making sure preventive and treatment plans meet the needs of the patient and prepare direct caregivers to participate as part of the health care team.[10,53,54]

Importantly, providers need to consider an onset of frailty at a younger age than the general population.[6] While there is no one universally accepted definitions of frailty, there are common elements that include a distinction from a disability, increased vulnerability, and intertwined with the social determinants of health, biology and some correlation with age.[55] Frail individuals are at higher risk of adverse events and poor outcomes of care.[56] While those who are most likely to be highly dependent and frail are of advanced age (ie, 80, 90+ years), for those with IDD this level of frailty could occur at 40 years of age or even younger due to accelerated aging.[6] Individuals with IDD and chronic disease have higher rates of pre-frailty and frailty than the general population.[55,56]

A consensus statement examines best practices to support individuals with IDD in pre-frailty and as they become frail (**Box 2**). To support aging individuals with IDD, there must be an increased awareness of the needs that come with increasing frailty and appropriate planning to meet those needs.[57] This extends oral health needs. The tenets posed in their consensus makes application of The Seattle Care Pathway (SCP) or Lucerne Pathway (Lucerne) approaches even more prescient given they are evidence-based approaches to oral health care and treatment planning focused on level of dependence rather than age.[53] This also applies to individuals with IDD, through the lens of conditions and diseases commonly associated with aging that may compound pre-existing issues of dependence.

Importantly this consensus suggests that pre-frailty and frailty can be reversed or stabilized.[55] Treatment planning schemas such as SCP and Lucerne recommend primarily preventive and palliative care in the most dependent stages. These philosophies may be aspirational in that they want adults to reach old age with their dentition intact and a healthy oral cavity and recommend oral health providers focus on prevention and palliative needs. The reality for many patients in a frail or dependent state is that they require more than preventive or palliative care to avoid acute conditions. The oral health status of this population is a result of all the risks to their oral health including their health conditions and their high dependence on others.[10,53] According to this consensus statement, their state of frailty is not definitive. As such it cannot be the only factor in determining appropriateness of care. Further, even if patients are aging in place we must also consider where this is occurring. The level of dependence is determined by whether they have access to a dental office/clinic or whether a provider can come to them for treatment. As needs change over time, whether they live at home or in a residential setting, an individual may require providers who can provide care in a dental office, a day center, another health care facility and/or at home.[54] A team of dental providers, dentists, hygienists, dental therapists, and assistants can be employed to best meet their needs.[35,47] Dental providers who can function as part of an inter-professional team and in a variety of clinical settings will be best prepared to care for individuals with increasing complexity of care. Even those

---

Box 2
Seven recommendations for a person-centered approach to planning and aging in place for individuals with IDD, International Expert Panel Recommendations[57,a]

1. Earlier consideration of frailty than in the general population

2. Improvement and maintenance as viable goals

3. Inter-sectoral collaboration to coordinate comprehensive multi-disciplinary assessments and actions

4. Safety as a priority

5. Planning for the future

6. Recognition of the needs of formal and informal caregivers

7. Acknowledgment the current evidence base is lacking and requires more investigation.

[a] The panel acknowledges that their consensus is the work of experts and that direct input from individuals with IDD themselves and their caregivers is needed.

with the most complex needs can benefit from patient centered care that does not wrongly assume an inability to receive or benefit from oral health care, based on disability or dependence alone. And their dental home does not have to be restricted to a traditional structure as many have come to know for the practice of dentistry.[54]

SUMMARY

Adults with IDD face a new intersectionality as they age. Many have challenged ablest stereotypes to gain and maintain their independence. Those who have had the benefit of oral health care often had to fit into spaces and respond to circumstances that were not designed to capitalize on their abilities, compromising outcomes. As they experience accelerated aging, fitting into these predetermined spaces can present even greater challenges. Carefully assessing the dental history that follows them and assessing the new risks to oral health from accelerated aging, disease, medications, and dependence on others is required to create preventive and treatment plans that are appropriate to each individual's needs. Understanding the transitions that lay ahead of them and their caregiver and the support structures that are in place or needed will come from an inter-professional approach to patient care. The oral health profession needs to take oral health care to those who cannot come to practitioners and thus improve access and experience when they demonstrate inclusivity toward marginalized populations and communities. Further advocating for resources that reduce disparities in oral health care are paramount to the inclusion of oral health care into the broader health care system and ensuring that adults of all ages and abilities have a dental home that is accessible to them so that they can age with the comfort and dignity that good oral health can provide.

CLINICS CARE POINTS

- The age of onset of chronic diseases commonly associated with older adults, is in younger ages for those with IDD.
- Attention to environments that support those with developmental and acquired disabilities promotes inclusivity.
- Good quality of life and positive treatment outcomes are possible for individuals at any age or stage of dependence.
- Significant systemic financial barriers exist for individuals with developmental and acquired disabilities, some of which are exacerbated in later years by a lack of coordinated care and resources for oral health care for adults.
- For individuals with increasing dependence or frailty, transitions in caregiving and residence will require additional consideration for inclusion in dental treatment planning and prevention.

DISCLOSURE

The authors have no conflicts of interest to disclose.

REFERENCES

1. Tinglin CC. Adults with intellectual and developmental disabilities: a unique population. Today's Geriatric Medicine 2013;6(3):22. Available at: https://www.

todaysgeriatricmedicine.com/archive/050613p22.shtml. Accessed June 11, 2024.

2. Parens E. Choosing flourishing: toward a more "binocular" way of thinking about disability. Kennedy Inst Ethics J 2017;27(2):135–50. https://doi.org/10.1353/ken. 2017.0013.

3. Centers for Disease Control and Prevention. Disability Impacts All of Us. 2023. Available at: https://www.cdc.gov/ncbddd/disabilityandhealth/infographic-disability-impacts-all.html. Accessed March 22, 2024.

4. Caplan Z. U.S. Older Population Grew from 2010 to 2020 at Fastest Rate Since 1880 to 1890. 2023. Available at: https://www.census.gov/library/stories/2023/05/2020-census-united-states-older-population-grew.html. Accessed June 11, 2024.

5. Lamb E. Disability and age studies. In: Reynolds JM, Wieseler C, editors. The Disability Bioethics Reader. New York: Routledge; 2022. p. 170–9.

6. Bradley VJ, Hiersteiner D, Li H, et al. What do NCI data tell us about the characteristics and outcomes of older adults with IDD? Developmental Disabilities Network J 2020;1(1):Article 6. https://doi.org/10.26077/esw0-2h31. Available at: https://digitalcommons.usu.edu/ddnj/vol1/iss1/6. Accessed June 11, 2024.

7. 2008-2017 U.S. Multiple cause-of-death mortality files, national vital statistics system. Available at: https://www.cdc.gov/nchs/nvss/mortality_public_use_data. htm. Accessed June 10, 2024.

8. Forrester SN, Zmora R, Schreiner PJ, et al. Accelerated aging: a marker for social factors resulting in cardiovascular events? SSM Popul Health 2021;13:100733.

9. Landes SD, Stevens JD, Turk MA. Cause of death in adults with intellectual disability in the United States. J Intellect Disabil Res 2021;65(1):47–59.

10. Chávez EM, Wong LM, Subar P, et al. Dental care for geriatric and special needs populations. Dent Clin North Am 2018;62(2):245–67.

11. Carmeli E, Imam B. Health promotion and disease prevention strategies in older adults with intellectual and developmental disabilities. Front Public Health 2014; 2:31.

12. Carmeli E, Ayalon M, Barchad S, et al. Isokinetic leg strength of institutionalized older adults with mental retardation with and without Down's syndrome. J Strength Cond Res 2002;16(2):316–20.

13. Molton IR, Goetz MC, Jensen MP, et al. Evidence for "accelerated aging" in older adults with disability? JAGS 2012;60(S4):239.

14. Pitts A. Disability Bioethics and Race. In: Reynolds JM, Wieseler C, editors. The disability bioethics reader. New York: Routledge; 2022. p. 235–42.

15. Linton S. Claiming Disability: Knowledge and Identity. New York: New York University Press; 1996.

16. Wendell S. The Rejected Body: Feminist Philosophical Reflections on Disability. New York: Routledge; 1996.

17. Reynolds JM. The extended body: on aging, disability, and well-being. Hastings Cent Rep 2018;48(Suppl 3):S31–6.

18. Rowe JW, Kahn RL. Successful aging. Gerontol 1997 Aug;37(4):433–40.

19. Gibbons HM, Owen R, Heller T. Perceptions of health and healthcare of people with intellectual and developmental disabilities in Medicaid managed care. Intellect Dev Disabil 2016;54(2):94–105.

20. Price M. The bodymind problem and the possibilities of pain. Hypatia 2015;30(1): 268–84.

21. Albrecht G, Devlieger P. The disability paradox: high quality of life against all odds. Soc Sci Med 1999;48:977–88.

22. Amundson R. Disability, Ideology, and Quality of life: A Bias in Biomedical Ethics. In: Wasserman D, Bickenbach J, Wachbroit R, editors. Quality of Life and human difference: genetic testing, health care, and disability. Cambridge studies in philosophy and public policy. Cambridge, England: Cambridge University Press; 2005. p. 101–24.

23. Nosek MA. Personal assistance: its effect on the long-term health of a rehabilitation hospital population. Arch Phys Med Rehabil 1993;74(2):127–32.

24. Silvers A. Predicting Genetic Disability While Commodifying Health. In: Wasserman D, Bickenbach J, Wachbroit R, editors. Quality of Life and human difference: genetic testing, health care, and disability. Cambridge studies in philosophy and public policy. Cambridge University Press; 2005. p. 43–66.

25. Campbell SM, Stramondo JA. The complicated relationship of disability and well being. Kennedy Inst Ethics J 2017;27(2):151–84.

26. Americans with Disabilities Act of 1990, as amended. Available at: https://www.ada.gov/law-and-regs/ada/. Accessed June 11, 2024.

27. Iezzoni LI, Rao SR, Ressalam J, et al. Physicians' perceptions of people with disability and their health care. Health Aff (Millwood) 2021;40(2):297–306.

28. Iezzoni L, O'Day B. More than Ramps: a Guide to Improving Health Care Quality and Access for People With Disabilities. New York: Oxford University Press; 2006. p. 101–2.

29. Burke TB. Bioethics and Deaf Community. In: Reynolds JM, Wieseler C, editors. The disability bioethics reader. New York: Routledge; 2022. p. 243–52.

30. Reiheld A. Methods of Bioethics. In: Reynolds JM, Wieseler C, editors. The disability bioethics reader. New York: Routledge; 2022. p. 50–60.

31. Schroer JW, Bain Z. "The Message is in the Microaggression: Epistemic Oppression at the Intersection of Disability and Race". In: Freeman L, Schroer JW, editors. Microaggressions and philosophy. New York: Routledge; 2020. p. 226–50.

32. Anders PL, Davis EL. Oral health of patients with intellectual disabilities: a systematic review. Spec Care Dentist 2010;30(3):110–7.

33. Wilson NJ, Lin Z, Villarosa A, et al. Oral health status and reported oral health problems in people with intellectual disability: a literature review. JIDD 2018; 44(3):292–304.

34. Morgan JP, Minihan PM, Stark PC, et al. The oral health status of 4,732 adults with intellectual and developmental disabilities. J Am Dent Assoc 2012;143(8): 838–46.

35. Glassman P. New models for improving oral health for people with special needs. J Calif Dent Assoc 2005;33(8):625–33.

36. Ettinger RL. Meeting oral health needs to promote the wellbeing of the geriatric population: educational research issues. J Dent Educ 2010;74(1):29–35.

37. Minihan PM. Aging in adults with developmental disabilities. In: Arenson C, Busby-Whitehead J, Brummel-Smith K, et al, editors. Reichel's care of the elderly. 6th edition. New York City: Cambridge University Press; 2009. p. 210–20.

38. U.S. Department of Health and Human Services. Oral Health in America: A Report of the Surgeon General. Rockville, MD: U.S. Department of Health and Human Services, National Institute of Dental and Craniofacial Research, National Institutes of Health, 2000.

39. Office of the Surgeon General; National Institute of Child Health and Human Development Centers for Disease Control and Prevention. Closing the gap: a national blueprint to improve the health of persons with mental retardation. Washington: U.S. Department of Health and Human Services; 2002.

40. U.S. Department of Health and Human Services. The Surgeon General's Call to Action to Improve the Health and Wellness of Persons with Disabilities. Rockville, MD: U.S. Department of Health and Human Services, Office of the Surgeon General, 2005.
41. Bridgman AM, Wilson MA. The treatment of adult patients with a mental disability, part 1: consent and duty. Br Dent J 2000;189(2):66–8.
42. Wilson NJ, Lin Z, Villarosa A, et al. Countering the poor oral health of people with intellectual and developmental disability: a scoping literature review. BMC Publ Health 2019;19(1):1530.
43. Cohen W, Rose LF, Minsk L. The periodontal–medical risk relationship. Compend Contin Educ Dent 2001;22(2 Spec No):7–11.
44. Walls AW, Steele JG. Geriatric oral health issues in the United Kingdom. Int Dent J 2001;51(3 Suppl):183–7.
45. Alves NS, Gavina VP, Cortellazzi KL, et al. Analysis of clinical, demographic, socioeconomic, and psychosocial determinants of quality of life of persons with intellectual disability: a cross-sectional study. Spec Care Dentist 2016;36(6): 307–14.
46. Coyle CE, Putman M, Kramer J, et al. The role of aging and disability resource centers in serving adults aging with intellectual disabilities and their families: findings from seven states. J Aging Soc Policy 2016;28(1):1–14.
47. National Institutes of Health. Oral health in America challenges and opportunities, an executive summary. Available at: https://www.nidcr.nih.gov/sites/default/files/2021-12/Oral-Health-in-America-Executive-Summary.pdf. Accessed June 10, 2024.
48. Medicare dental coverage. Available at: https://www.cms.gov/medicare/coverage/dental. Accessed June 10, 2024.
49. Heller T, Scott HM, Janicki MP. Pre-summit workgroup on caregiving and intellectual/developmental disabilities. Caregiving, intellectual disability, and dementia: report of the summit workgroup on caregiving and intellectual and developmental disabilities. Alzheimers Dement (NY) 2018;4:272–82.
50. Understanding aging for individuals with intellectual and developmental disabilities HCBS conference. Available at: https://na.eventscloud.com/file_uploads/9cf35c695e7cdd60405b04531fa7dc9f_2015HCBSSessionAgingIDDWednesday Sept23_4.15p.m.GeorgetownEast.pdf. Accessed June 10, 2024.
51. Lee CE, Burke MM, Arnold CK, et al. Compound sibling caregivers of individuals with intellectual and developmental disabilities. J Appl Res Intellect Disabil 2020; 33(5):1069–79.
52. Lee CE, Burke MM, Perkins EA. Compound caregiving: toward a research agenda. Intellect Dev Disabil 2022;60(1):66–79.
53. Pretty IA, Ellwood RP, Lo E, et al. The Seattle Care Pathway for securing oral health in older patients. Gerodontology 2014;31(s1):77–87.
54. Ghezzi EM, Fisher MM. Strategies for oral health care practitioners to manage older adults through care-setting transitions. J Calif Dent Assoc 2019;47(4): 235–45.
55. McKenzie K, Martin L, Ouellette-Kuntz H. Frailty and intellectual and developmental disabilities: a scoping review. Can Geriatr J 2016;19(3):103–12.
56. Lin SY, Tseng HC. Short-term changes of frailty in prematurely aging adults with intellectual disability. Intellect Dev Disabil 2022;60(1):57–65.
57. Ouellette-Kuntz H, Martin L, Burke E, et al. How best to support individuals with IDD as they become frail: development of a consensus statement. J Appl Res Intellect Disabil 2019;32(1):35–42.

Sex and Gender Health Education Tenets
An Essential Paradigm for Inclusivity in Dentistry

Joanne L. Prasad, DDS, MPH[a,b,]*, Mary K. Rojek, PhD[c],
Sara C. Gordon, DDS, MS[d],
Linda M. Kaste, DDS, MS, PhD, FAADOCR, FICD[e],
Leslie R. Halpern, DDS, MD, PhD, MPH, FICD[f]

KEYWORDS

• Sex • Gender • Oral health • Dental education • Competencies • Inclusivity • Bias

KEY POINTS

- Sex and gender are integral to person-centered care.
- Interprofessional sex and gender health tenets (competencies) were recently published for health sciences education and are applied here for dentistry.
- Oral health curricula should ensure that graduates understand sex and gender differences and can apply this knowledge to the comprehensive care of patients.
- Evidence-based care depends on health sciences research including sex and gender considerations.
- Sex and gender health advocacy will help improve health outcomes and reduce health disparities.

[a] Department of Oral and Craniofacial Sciences, University of Pittsburgh School of Dental Medicine, 3501 Terrace Street, G-133 Salk Annex, Pittsburgh, PA 15261, USA; [b] Department of Diagnostic Sciences, University of Pittsburgh School of Dental Medicine, 3501 Terrace Street, G-133 Salk Annex, Pittsburgh, PA 15261, USA; [c] University of South Carolina School of Medicine Greenville, 607 Grove Road, Greenville, SC 29605, USA; [d] Department of Oral Medicine, School of Dentistry, University of Washington, 1959 Northeast Pacific Street, HSB B-530F, Box 357480, Seattle, WA 98195-7480, USA; [e] Department of Oral Biology, University of Illinois Chicago, 801 South Paulina Street, MC 690, Chicago, IL 60612, USA; [f] Oral and Maxillofacial Surgery Residency, New York Medical College, 40 Sunshine Cottage Road, Valhalla, NY 10595, USA
* Corresponding author. Department of Oral and Craniofacial Sciences, University of Pittsburgh School of Dental Medicine, 3501 Terrace Street, G-133 Salk Annex, Pittsburgh, PA 15261.
E-mail address: jlp92@pitt.edu

Dent Clin N Am 69 (2025) 115–130
https://doi.org/10.1016/j.cden.2024.08.008
dental.theclinics.com

INTRODUCTION
Sex, Gender, and Health

Sex and gender are essential components of oral and systemic health. Adopting a sex and gender lens is paramount in providing person-centered and evidence-based care. "Sex" (female, male, intersex, or non-dichotomous sex) is a biologic variable determined by the presence and/or combination of sex chromosomes, sex hormones, and reproductive organs. A person's sex directly impacts the function of their cells and has broad physiologic and pathophysiologic implications relevant to all organ systems.[1] "Gender" (man, woman, transgender, and nonbinary genders) is a sociocultural spectrum associated with certain roles, habits and behaviors, identities, and power relations[2,3] that occur in a social, cultural, and historic context. These may influence the risk of disease and a person's interactions with the health care system. The interaction between biologic sex and sociocultural gender has an impact on health.

Evolution of Sex and Gender in Dental Education

Key events in the development of sex and gender core educational competency statements, or "tenets," that apply to all health profession programs are outlined in **Fig. 1**.

In the early 1990s, increased awareness of sex differences in health and disease propelled the incorporation of women's health issues into research and clinical practice.[4] In 1996, the US Department of Health and Human Services concluded that all health professionals should competently provide care to women across the life span.[5] In response, a 1997 dental curricular survey explored topics in women's health, serving as the impetus for the subsequent survey report and for a discussion of women's oral health in a 2001 *Dental Clinics of North America (DCNA)* publication.[6,7] A second comprehensive dental curricular survey on closely parallel subject areas followed over a decade later, in 2011 (**Box 1**).[8] It indicated that gender-related topics were incorporated into dental curricula at many institutions. Participants agreed the information was important but that faculty needed resources and guidelines on content, sequencing, and/or assessment of these topics. The report recommended establishing national educational and fellowship programs and resources related to women's health; incorporating "clinical simulations" for teaching women's health topics into dental curricula; promoting interprofessional dialogue to address sex and gender factors in health and disease; and developing core competencies related to sex and gender health (SGH). A second *DCNA* issue focused on these emerging perspectives.[9]

A series of interprofessional SGH Education Summits in 2015, 2018, 2020, and 2021 broadened the approach from a focus on women to include all genders and sexes. At the 2020 SGH Education Summit, facilitated discussion groups composed of members representing health disciplines including dentistry drafted four interprofessional SGH core competency statements, or "tenets," for educational programs in all health professions. A smaller interprofessional working group revised, finalized, and published the tenets (**Box 2**).[10]

DISCUSSION: THE SEX AND GENDER HEALTH EDUCATION TENETS

The integration of SGH tenets in dental education will help dental schools incorporate SGH topics into dental curricula. This will establish best practices and calibration of education, support interprofessional collaboration, improve patient care, reduce bias, and advance inclusivity. Each tenet is outlined and discussed later, along with some applications for dentistry. Exhaustive discussion of all SGH topics is well beyond the scope of this article, so we recommend reviewing prior and emerging publications

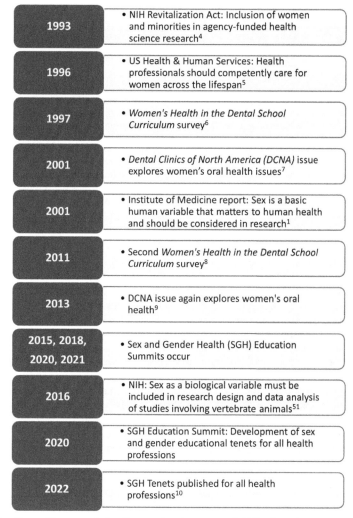

1993	• NIH Revitalization Act: Inclusion of women and minorities in agency-funded health science research[4]
1996	• US Health & Human Services: Health professionals should competently care for women across the lifespan[5]
1997	• *Women's Health in the Dental School Curriculum* survey[6]
2001	• *Dental Clinics of North America (DCNA)* issue explores women's oral health issues[7]
2001	• Institute of Medicine report: Sex is a basic human variable that matters to human health and should be considered in research[1]
2011	• Second *Women's Health in the Dental School Curriculum* survey[8]
2013	• DCNA issue again explores women's oral health[9]
2015, 2018, 2020, 2021	• Sex and Gender Health (SGH) Education Summits occur
2016	• NIH: Sex as a biological variable must be included in research design and data analysis of studies involving vertebrate animals[51]
2020	• SGH Education Summit: Development of sex and gender educational tenets for all health professions
2022	• SGH Tenets published for all health professions[10]

Fig. 1. Timeline of key events leading to development of SGH education tenets.

on this subject to further guide incorporation of SGH in dental education and practice.[7–9,11,12]

Tenet 1: Demonstrate Knowledge of Sex and Gender Health

The intent of Tenet 1 is summarized in **Box 3**.

Biomedical, behavioral, and clinical courses should highlight diseases and conditions with a sex and/or gender prevalence or differences in clinical presentation, treatment, or prognosis. This should accompany instruction related to screening, evaluation, risk assessment, diagnosis, treatment, health promotion, and disease prevention strategies. Some examples include eating disorders, head and neck cancer, osteoporosis, sleep apnea, temporomandibular disorders, autoimmune diseases, and developmental anomalies. Pregnancy and prenatal care should also be addressed. Additional examples are provided in **Table 1**.

Box 1
Survey on women's health in dental school curriculum: comparison of 1999 and 2011 topic areas

1997 Survey Topic Areas[6]	2011 Survey Topic Areas[8]
General Social Themes and Gender	General Themes
Biological and Basic Science Considerations	Biological Considerations
Developmental and Psychological Themes	Developmental and Social Issues
Health Behavior and Health Promotion	Approaches to Health Behavior/Health Promotion in Women
Sexual and Reproductive Function	Sexual and Reproductive Function
Selected Conditions Prevalent in Women	Etiology, Prevalence, Course Treatment, and Prevention of Particular Conditions/Disorders in Women
Impact of Medications	Impact of the Use of Medications
History, Physical Examination, and Communication Skills	History, Physical Examination, and Patient Communication Skills
Selected Topics of Concern to Women	N/A

The remainder of this section on Tenet 1 will focus on a discussion of sex and gender differences in the underlying mechanisms of pain and disease. Currently, little information exists in the scientific literature on the effects of exogenous hormones on pain and disease in transgender persons.

Sexual dimorphism in pain mechanisms

Pain is commonly encountered in dental practice. Female individuals tend to be more sensitive to pain (lower pain threshold and tolerance) and experience pain more intensely than male individuals.[13] Physiologic mechanisms underlying pain in male individuals are significantly different than those producing pain in female individuals.[13–18] Estrogen and androgen receptors are found on many cells including neurons, glial cells, and immune cells. Sex hormones influence pain by binding to those receptors.[19] Tissue-specific co-regulating proteins are sometimes involved. In general, testosterone appears to have antinociceptive effects, whereas the effects of estrogen and progesterone on pain vary and are less clear. For premenopausal female individuals, pain intensity may also parallel normal fluctuations in estrogen and progesterone during the menstrual cycle.[13] Prolactin, which has numerous functions beyond lactation, is also linked to sex differences in pain. Estrogen promotes expression of prolactin receptor isoforms that are linked with pain.[20]

Immune cells play an important role in pain and studies show sex differences in immune modulation of pain.[13,16,17] Macrophages can induce pain or increase pain sensitivity via the release of proinflammatory cytokines. Microglia in the spinal cord increase pain in male mice but not females through testosterone-dependent binding of a

Box 2
Sex and gender health education tenets[10]

Tenet 1: *Demonstrate knowledge of sex and gender health.*

Tenet 2: *Evaluate literature and the conduct of research for incorporation of sex and gender.*

Tenet 3: *Incorporate sex and gender considerations into decision-making.*

Tenet 4: *Demonstrate patient advocacy with respect to sex and gender.*

Box 3
Tenet 1: demonstrate knowledge of sex and gender health[10]

Dental practitioners should be able to
- Define sex and gender as variables that impact health and influence risk for disease at all stages of life.
- Describe and explain sex differences and the interaction between sex and gender in anatomy, physiology, and pathophysiology.
- Identify and describe psychosocial factors and behaviors that influence the risk of disease or health outcomes.

---

lipopolysaccharide ligand to its toll-like receptor 4 (TLR4).[21–23] TLR4 is linked to chronic pain and sepsis in male individuals, but not in female individuals. In female individuals, pain is preferentially modulated by a subset of helper T cells with proinflammatory properties (CD4+ Th1).[16,17] Female individuals exhibit a predominance of CD4+ Th1 T cells, whereas male individuals show higher levels of anti-inflammatory CD4+ Th2 T cells. These differences appear to be mediated by estrogen and progesterone levels in female individuals and testosterone in male individuals.[24]

Sex hormones influence the stress-induced analgesia (SIA) system, a centrally mediated innate defensive mechanism that suppresses pain in response to a stressful stimulus. It involves opioid and glutamate receptors as well as neurotransmitters such as beta-endorphin and results in the inhibition of descending pain pathways.[25] The N-methyl-D-aspartate (NMDA) glutamate receptor is involved in activation of SIA in male individuals but not female individuals. However, when estrogen production is significantly reduced, female individuals "switch" to the NMDA pathway. Exposure to testosterone during the neonatal period appears critical to this sex difference. A female-specific SIA pathway involves the melanocortin-1 receptor (MC1R), widely expressed in melanocytes and glial cells of the brain. Mutations that render MC1R nonfunctional also result in a "switch" to the NMDA system.[15,17]

Gender and pain
Chronic pain (CP), a leading cause of disability worldwide, affects 20% of adults. Women suffer from CP conditions at higher rates than men.[26] Biologic differences affect how pain is experienced, but the influence of sociocultural, psychological, and gender factors on pain sensitivity, experience, coping, and reporting cannot be overlooked.[1,27] In women who have experienced traumatic life events such as violence and abuse, the emotional context of pain and stress can lead to modifications in nervous, endocrine, and immune function, increased sensitivity to nociceptive stimuli, and greater susceptibility to CP conditions.[28]

For example, symptomatic temporomandibular disorders (TMDs) are reported disproportionally by women.[29,30] Unraveling the relative contributions of sex and gender to symptomatic TMD is complex. Genetic predisposition has been linked to polymorphisms in certain pain-related genes.[31] Estrogen receptors (ERs) abound in the temporomandibular joint, and polymorphisms in ER-alpha are associated with an increased risk of TMD.[32] Additionally, blockage of ERs in synovial cells appears to inhibit cartilage and bone destruction in temporomandibular joint osteoarthritis.[33] Estrogen levels also may explain the higher prevalence of TMD in women of reproductive years and a 30% increase in TMD in women taking estrogen-containing oral contraceptives.[34,35]

Women are more likely to seek medical care than men. This could contribute to sex and gender disparities in the reported prevalence of some painful conditions including TMD.[36] Depending on culture-specific gender roles and expectations, women may be

Table 1
Examples of oral pathologic conditions with a marked sex/gender predilection

Male Predominant Oral Pathologic Conditions and Lesions	Male: Female Ratio
Blastomycosis	9:1
Kaposi sarcoma	9:1
Lymphatic malformations	2:1
Nasopharyngeal angiofibroma	Almost exclusively in male individuals
Necrotizing sialometaplasia	Approaching 2:1
Oral leukoplakia	4:1
Oral squamous cell carcinoma	2.7:1
Orthokeratinized odontogenic cyst	2.6:1
Paracoccidioidomycosis	13:1
Stafne bone defect	8:1–9:1
Warthin tumor	10:1

Female Predominant Oral Pathologic Conditions and Lesions	Female: Male Ratio
Proliferative Verrucous Leukoplakia	4:1
Sjögren syndrome	9:1–20:1[41]
Polymorphous low-grade adenocarcinoma	2:1
Oral focal mucinosis	2:1
Granular cell tumor	3:1
Congenital epulis	9:1
Alveolar soft-part sarcoma	2:1
Rheumatoid arthritis	2:1–3:1
Focal osteoporotic bone marrow defect	3:1
Periapical cemento-osseous dysplasia	10:1–14:1
Florid cemento-osseous dysplasia	9:1
Adenomatoid odontogenic tumor	2:1
Mucous membrane pemphigoid	2:1
Systemic lupus erythematosus	10:1
Hyperthyroidism (Grave's disease)	5:1–10:1
Hyperparathyroidism	2:1–4:1
Trigeminal neuralgia	3:1
Giant cell arteritis	2:1–3:1

As reported in the dental education textbook: Neville BW, Damm DD, Allen CM, and Chi AC. Oral and Maxillofacial Pathology. 5th edition. 2024. Elsevier.[77]

more likely to report and outwardly express pain.[37,38] Coping mechanisms may also differ between men and women and can impact the CP experience.[38] These psychosociocultural factors may also alter the pain experience itself.

The X chromosome: X-linked and autoimmune disorders
Most human cells have 46 chromosomes, including two sex chromosomes (XX for females/XY for males). In euploid female individuals, one of the two X chromosomes is randomly inactivated ("silenced") during early embryologic development. The silencing process usually results in a relatively equal distribution of maternal versus paternal X chromosomes; however, skewing toward one allele may occur. The

inactivation process is also imperfect, and some genes on the inactivated chromosome may "escape" silencing.[39] These epigenetic phenomena may partially account for female-predominant diseases.[40]

The Y chromosome contains 106 active protein-coding genes; many primarily involved in male sex determination and development.[41] In contrast, the X chromosome contains 1098 active, protein-coding genes,[42] with a wide array of potential gene products and functions. Sex-linked disorders occur when a mutated gene implicated in a particular disease is located on the X or Y chromosome. Given the large number of genes located on the X chromosome, most sex-linked disorders are X linked. X-linked recessive disorders, such as hemophilia A and B, primarily affect male offspring, although female offspring may also be affected in rare cases, when skewing or gene activation imbalances exist.

Sex chromosomes also appear to be responsible for fundamental physiologic differences that influence the risk of autoimmune diseases. The X chromosome holds many immune genes, which may help explain the greater prevalence of autoimmune disorders among female individuals.[40] While the exact mechanism is not entirely clear, extreme skewing and activation of "escaped" genes are plausible explanations. Sjögren's syndrome, up to 20 times more common in women, is a useful model to study the role of X chromosome genes such as toll-like receptor 7 (immune response initiation), CD40 ligand (B cell activation), C-X-C motif chemokine receptor (chemokine expression), and interleukin-1 receptor associated kinase (proinflammatory pathways activation).[40] Other autoimmune diseases with a strong female predilection include systemic lupus erythematosus, systemic sclerosis, rheumatoid arthritis, autoimmune thyroiditis, Grave's disease, and multiple sclerosis.

Sex differences in immunity

Female individuals exhibit a more vigorous immune response to infections and vaccination, which has been linked to sex hormones.[43] Testosterone in male individuals is generally anti-inflammatory as it appears to inhibit the differentiation of B cells and helper T cells and the release of cytokines from T cells.[17,44–46] This may explain both the lower prevalence of autoimmune disorders and also the more attenuated immune response to vaccination and infection in male individuals. In contrast, estrogen's effects on immune cells are typically but not always proinflammatory. Estrogen directly enhances the function of several immune cells, such as T cells, natural killer cells, and macrophages. Progesterone's effects on immune function are less studied; however, it appears to reduce inflammation.

Bone health

Bone is formed, resorbed, and maintained by osteoblasts, osteoclasts, and osteocytes, respectively. In female individuals, bone mass and bone density sharply decrease following menopause. Nearly 20% of female individuals aged over 50 years are diagnosed with osteoporosis and more than 50% show low bone mass.[47] Estrogen inhibits osteoblast expression of a ligand that activates osteoclasts (receptor activator of nuclear factor kappa B ligand [RANKL]).[48] When estrogen levels drop after menopause, RANKL expression increases. In contrast, testosterone promotes bone mineral density through incompletely understood mechanisms.[49,50] The risk of medication-related osteonecrosis of the jaws is elevated in patients taking bisphosphonates and/or other antiresorptive agents for the management of osteoporosis.

Tenet 2: Evaluate Literature and the Conduct of Research for Incorporation of Sex and Gender

The intent of Tenet 2 is summarized in **Box 4**.

> **Box 4**
> **Tenet 2: evaluate literature and conduct of research for incorporation of sex and gender[10]**
> Dental practitioners should be able to
> - Use a sex and gender lens to critically evaluate the research literature.
> - Find evidence to support treatment decisions that consider sex and gender and proceed with caution when there is no evidence.
> - Incorporate or consider sex and gender in the design, conduct, analysis, and reporting of research.

Dental curricula should emphasize the importance of sex and gender in health sciences research and in evidence-based dentistry.

The traditional understanding of health and disease was based primarily on a male model. Women have been historically excluded or underrepresented in biomedical and health sciences research. Research that does consider sex and gender in health, disease, and medicine clearly demonstrates significant differences across many biomedical and clinical sciences domains. In 1993, the National Institutes of Health (NIH) Revitalization Act became US law, establishing guidelines to include women and minorities in agency-funded health science research.[4] A 2001 Institute of Medicine report concluded that sex is a basic human variable that matters to human health and should be considered in the conduct of research.[1]

Until recently, animal studies were excluded from the NIH policy related to the inclusion of sex and gender in clinical research. In 2016, the NIH revised its policy to include a mandate to consider sex as a biologic variable in the design and data analysis of studies involving vertebrate animals.[51] Research designs that exclude one sex must provide "strong justification from the scientific literature, preliminary data, or other relevant considerations" for doing so. Results of any preclinical or clinical study that does not report the sex of the cell lines or subjects, does not include adequate numbers of male/men and female/women subjects, and/or does not disaggregate the data for analysis should be interpreted with caution, may not be generalizable, and may have limited clinical relevance.

Tenet 3: Incorporate Sex and Gender Considerations into Decision-Making

The intent of Tenet 3 is summarized in **Box 5**.

Sex and gender should be considered to optimize oral health for all persons.

Caries and periodontal disease

US studies indicate that men are more likely than women to exhibit periodontal disease-related attachment loss and probing depths greater than 3 mm, although a few older studies report a higher prevalence of periodontal disease in girls compared to boys. Studies indicate a higher prevalence of dental decay in women compared to men in the US population, although this difference may be linked to gender-based socioeconomic disparities.[52]

The relative contribution of biologic versus behavioral factors in the development of caries and periodontal disease is difficult to ascertain, but evidence suggests that diet, smoking, oral hygiene practices, health attitudes, and behaviors play roles.[53–55] Approaches to prevent disease and promote oral health should consider addressing gender-specific behaviors. For example, men are more likely to use tobacco and reportedly brush, floss, and visit the dentist less frequently than women. No evidence exists yet to recommend sex-specific therapies to address caries and periodontal disease, but gender-specific messaging about prevention may be useful.

> **Box 5**
> **Tenet 3: incorporate sex and gender considerations into decision-making**[10]
>
> Dental practitioners should be able to
> - Describe sex and gender as components of person-centered care.
> - Use a sex and gender lens when considering treatment options.
> - Use appropriate, evidence-based therapeutic approaches and health promotion strategies to optimize health outcomes.

Head and neck cancer

While head and neck cancers affect both men and women, research and epidemiologic studies show a higher incidence of oral, salivary gland, pharyngeal, and laryngeal cancers in men compared to women.[52] Behavioral risk factors for head and neck cancer include tobacco use, alcohol consumption, actinic damage, and infection with high-risk human papillomavirus. However, a higher prevalence of cancer has been reported in male individuals even after adjusting for such behavioral risk factors, suggesting that underlying biologic factors such as sex hormones may play a role in differences between the sexes.[56] In male individuals, androgens appear to increase the risk of cancer. In female individuals, use of oral contraceptives may be associated with an increased risk of head and neck cancer, while hormone replacement therapy after menopause may lower the risk.[56]

When a lesion appears clinically suspicious, clinicians should not rely heavily on prevalence data or social and behavioral risk factors in clinical decision-making, as this may lead to a false assumption that could delay diagnosis and treatment. Oral cancer can affect individuals with no known risk factors.

Sex-specific targeted therapies for head and neck cancer have not yet been developed. However, given the ongoing evolution of personalized medicine, treatment may eventually become sex specific. Currently, addressing behavioral risk factors may help reduce head and neck cancer in both sexes.

Tobacco use

Given the consequences of smoking tobacco on systemic and oral health, dental providers should be aware of sex and gender differences related to tobacco cessation strategies.[57,58] For example, while treatment with varenicline is effective in both men and women, research shows that men respond better to nicotine replacement therapy and bupropion than women. Tobacco is addictive and biologic differences related to addiction and nicotine-motivated behavior may have an impact on tobacco cessation.[59] Overall, women are less likely to quit smoking and are more likely to relapse. Perceived risks of smoking cessation, such as weight gain, may have a greater influence on motivation to quit in women compared to men. Use of tobacco tends to be more frequently linked to the setting and mood among women, reflecting another gender difference. Providers should consider such differences to maximize the chance of success.

Pregnancy

Dental providers may be reluctant to manage the oral health needs of gravid patients, fearing harm to the fetus. However, pregnant patients benefit from, and should receive, routine dental care. The American Dental Association policy on dental treatment during pregnancy states that "preventive, diagnostic, and restorative dental treatment to promote health and eliminate disease is safe throughout pregnancy and is effective in improving and maintaining the oral health of the mother and child."[60]

The risk of gingivitis and periodontal disease increases during pregnancy due to the stimulatory effects of gonadal hormones on vascular permeability and inflammatory mediators.[61] Nonsurgical periodontal therapy should be provided prenatally and throughout pregnancy to optimize periodontal health and minimize the risk of pregnancy-related complications.[62,63]

Gravid patients may also experience recurrent vomiting leading to dental erosion. Oral health providers should inquire about emesis and instruct affected patients to rinse with warm water and avoid toothbrushing for an hour after vomiting. In-office fluoride application should also be considered.

Dental radiographs are considered safe and should be performed as needed during pregnancy with appropriate shielding, although the dentist and patient may be most comfortable limiting their use to urgent conditions.[64] Acetaminophen is generally appropriate for pain while non-steroidal anti-inflammatory drugs such as ibuprofen should be avoided.[65] When indicated, antibiotics can also be prescribed, including penicillin, amoxicillin, cephalexin, and clindamycin. Lidocaine and prilocaine can be used safely but longer lasting anesthetics, such as mepivacaine and bupivacaine, should be avoided.[61]

Sex differences in pharmacokinetics and pharmacodynamics

In the past, drug trials did not include female subjects and/or did not adequately analyze and report sex differences. Significant differences such as gastric motility, enzyme activity, glomerular filtration rate, and body fat distribution can impact the absorption, distribution, metabolism, and elimination of drugs.[66] Drug-related adverse reactions are more common in women. Most drugs withdrawn from the market were associated with a greater risk of adverse events in women, including death.[67] Pharmacology courses in dental curricula should include a discussion of sex differences in pharmacokinetics and pharmacodynamics, particularly related to drugs used in dentistry. For example, enzymes involved in the metabolism of benzodiazepines, acetaminophen, and epinephrine are more active in male individuals than female individuals.

Sex differences in opioid analgesia should be considered in managing acute dental and postoperative pain. Male animals are generally more sensitive to the effects of opioid analgesics. The type of opioid may matter; female individuals appear to be more sensitive to mixed mu/kappa agonists.[68] These differences are likely related to sex differences in SIA mechanisms outlined previously and in the sex hormone sensitivity and density of opioid receptors at various sites.

Tenet 4: Demonstrate Patient Advocacy with Respect to Sex and Gender

The intent of Tenet 4 is summarized in **Box 6**.

Dental graduates must possess the interpersonal communication skills and values necessary to care for a sex and gender-diverse patient population and demonstrate patient advocacy with respect to sex and gender.

Person-centered care and patient education

Demonstrating patient advocacy requires appropriate foundational knowledge, skills, and values related to SGH. Clinicians must understand that sex and gender are both intersectional parts of all of their patient's social identities and relate to their social determinants of health. Clinicians must be competent in reviewing the scientific literature to make informed treatment decisions based on the unique needs, risks, and goals of their patients. They should be curious and espouse lifelong learning because new discoveries and therapies are likely to emerge from SGH research. Clinicians should also

---

Box 6
Tenet 4: demonstrate patient advocacy with respect to sex and gender[10]

Dental practitioners should be able to
- Ensure that sex and gender are integrated in education, in the provision of person-centered care, and in the conduct of research.
- Advocate for, inform, and enable a sex and gender-diverse population of patients to improve their health.
- Demonstrate respect for all persons in interpersonal communications.
- Create safe and welcoming spaces that will improve access to care.

---

be alert to potential sex and gender differences in responses to medications among their patients, even when such differences have not yet been reported in research findings.

Oral health care providers should also exercise vigilance with regard to sex-related and gender-related health risks, such as intimate partner violence, prevalence of certain diseases, and sleep apnea. Advocacy includes educating patients regarding their unique oral health risks and SGH emerging knowledge. Person-centered care should be enabling, so that patients can acquire the knowledge, skills, and confidence to assume positive self-care behaviors.

Bias and communication
Clinicians must be aware of their own potential biases as health providers. Doctor–patient gender concordance influences patient care and the flow and quality of communication between clinician and patient. For example, physicians are more likely to prescribe opioid analgesics to same-sex patients.[69] Doctor–patient gender concordance also influences the flow and quality of information and communication between a clinician and a patient. Exchanges between women clinicians and men patients are perceived as the most tense and least friendly. When the doctor is a man and the patient is a woman, there tends to be the least exchange of information, a focus on treatment at the expense of self-care, and conversations that are the least patient centered. However, when the clinician and patient are both men, there tends to be more conversation and exchange of information, discussion of social risk factors and self-management, and more comradery. Finally, encounters between clinicians and patients who are both women are the most patient centered, offer the most encouragement, and are associated with a greater bidirectional flow of information.[70,71] Attending to implicit biases that we all possess will help reduce disparities in health outcomes among patients.

Create a welcoming environment
Advocacy involves creating a clinical environment that feels safe and welcoming to patients. This is particularly important in addressing health disparities that affect lesbian, gay, bisexual, transgender, queer, and other sex and gender-diverse (LGBTQ+) populations.[72,73] While factors such as environmental exposures, behaviors, and socioeconomic circumstances likely contribute to such disparities, the impact of negative interactions with the health care system is also important to the health of LGBTQ+ communities. Discrimination caused by explicit or implicit biases, or even the expectation of discrimination, can create stress and a significant barrier to care. One study found that 43% of LGBTQ+ patients felt uncomfortable going to dental appointments and 34% believed they had been treated unfairly. Inclusive health care practices, particularly enabling patients to indicate their pronouns, were

associated with a higher level of comfort.[74] Another study found that a safe and welcoming environment had a significant impact on promoting a positive attitude toward dental providers and minimizing barriers to care. Providing separate selections for "sex at birth" and "gender identity" on the intake form, noting a person's chosen name in addition to their legal name, and displaying physical signs of inclusion, such as a rainbow flag, can help to make LGBTQ+ patients feel comfortable and welcomed.[75] A 2016 *DCNA* article provides an excellent review of oral health and overall health of LGBTQ+ communities, reviews definitions (which will continue to evolve), and offers a list of suggestions and useful resources to improve LGBTQ+ oral health care.[12]

To advocate for patients, oral health care providers must seek opportunities to develop and enhance their knowledge, skills, and values in providing culturally competent care to a diverse patient population. In this current issue of *DCNA*, Haley and Doubleday offer an in-depth discussion of inclusive language in dentistry.[76]

SUMMARY

The integration of sex and gender competencies into dental curricula is essential to promote inclusivity in dentistry, reduce bias, and improve patient outcomes. The 4 tenets discussed in this article and the information presented under each tenet provide dental educators with a framework for developing educational content and materials that will ensure safe and competent, person-centered and evidence-based care for all patients.

CLINICS CARE POINTS

> - Sex and gender are essential components of dental education and clinical practice.
> - Knowledge of sex and gender differences will improve detection, treatment, and prognosis of oral diseases (Tenet 1).
> - Clinicians should adopt a sex and gender lens to critically evaluate research and scientific literature to support treatment decisions (Tenet 2).
> - Considering a person's sex and gender will help ensure treatment and prevention approaches are appropriate and person-centered (Tenet 3).
> - Integrating knowledge of sex and gender differences into patient communication will improve doctor/patient relationships and quality of patient care (Tenet 4).

DISCLOSURES

The authors have no relevant financial or nonfinancial conflicts of interests to disclose that are relevant to the content of this article.

REFERENCES

1. Institute of Medicine. Exploring the biological contributions to human health: does sex matter? Washington, DC: The National Academies Press; 2001.
2. Madsen TE, Bourjeily G, Hasnain M, et al. Article commentary: sex- and gender-based medicine: the need for precise terminology. Gender and the Genome 2017;1(3):122–8.
3. Mauvais-Jarvis F, Bairey Merz N, Barnes PJ, et al. Sex and gender: modifiers of health, disease, and medicine. Lancet 2020;396(10250):565–82.

4. National Institutes of Health Revitalization Act of 1993. Title I: General Provisions Regarding title IV of Public Health Service Act §131 (1993). Available at: https://www.congress.gov/bill/103rd-congress/senate-bill/1/text. Accessed September 10, 2024.

5. Sumaya CV, Pinn VW, Blumenthal SJ. Women's health in the medical school curriculum: report of a survey and recommendations. Rockville, MD: U.S. Department of Health and Human Services, Health Resources and Services Administration; 1997.

6. Silverton S, Sinkford J, Inglehart M, et al. Women's health in the dental school curriculum: a report of a survey and recommendations. Rockville, MD: U.S. Department of Health and Human Services, Health Resources and Services Administration; 2000.

7. Studen-Pavlovich D, Ranalli DN. Evolution of women's oral health. Dent Clin North Am 2001;45(3):433–42, v.

8. Women's Health in the Dental School Curriculum 2012: survey report and recommendations. Bethesda, MD: U.S. Department of Health and Human Services, Health Resources and Services Administration, and National Institutes of Health Office of Research on Women's Health, 2012.

9. Halpern LR, Kaste LM, Briggs C, et al. Women's oral health: growing evidence for enhancing perspectives. Dent Clin North Am 2013;57(2):xv–xxviii.

10. Kling JM, Sleeper R, Chin EL, et al. Sex and gender health educational tenets: a report from the 2020 sex and gender health education summit. J Womens Health (Larchmt) 2022;31(7):905–10.

11. Sinkford JC, Valachovic RW, Harrison SG. Women's oral health: the evolving science. J Dent Educ 2008;72(2):131–4.

12. Russell S, More F. Addressing health disparities via coordination of care and interprofessional education: lesbian, gay, bisexual, and transgender health and oral health care. Dent Clin North Am 2016;60(4):891–906.

13. Mogil JS. Sex differences in pain and pain inhibition: multiple explanations of a controversial phenomenon. Nat Rev Neurosci 2012;13(12):859–66.

14. Greenspan JD, Craft RM, LeResche L, et al. Studying sex and gender differences in pain and analgesia: a consensus report. Pain 2007;132(Suppl 1):S26–45.

15. Craft RM, Mogil JS, Aloisi AM. Sex differences in pain and analgesia: the role of gonadal hormones. Eur J Pain 2004;8(5):397–411.

16. Rosen S, Ham B, Mogil JS. Sex differences in neuroimmunity and pain. J Neurosci Res 2017;95(1–2):500–8.

17. Sorge RE, Totsch SK. Sex differences in pain. J Neurosci Res 2017;95(6):1271–81.

18. Bartley EJ, Fillingim RB. Sex differences in pain: a brief review of clinical and experimental findings. Br J Anaesth 2013;111(1):52–8.

19. Katzenellenbogen BS, Katzenellenbogen JA. Estrogen receptor transcription and transactivation: estrogen receptor alpha and estrogen receptor beta: regulation by selective estrogen receptor modulators and importance in breast cancer. Breast Cancer Res 2000;2(5):335–44.

20. Chen Y, Navratilova E, Dodick DW, et al. An emerging role for prolactin in female-selective pain. Trends Neurosci 2020;43(8):635–48.

21. Sorge RE, LaCroix-Fralish ML, Tuttle AH, et al. Spinal cord Toll-like receptor 4 mediates inflammatory and neuropathic hypersensitivity in male but not female mice. J Neurosci 2011;31(43):15450–4.

22. Sorge RE, Mapplebeck JC, Rosen S, et al. Different immune cells mediate mechanical pain hypersensitivity in male and female mice. Nat Neurosci 2015;18(8):1081–3.

23. Beutler B, Poltorak A. The sole gateway to endotoxin response: how LPS was identified as Tlr4, and its role in innate immunity. Drug Metab Dispos 2001;29(4 Pt 2):474–8.

24. Amadori A, Zamarchi R, De Silvestro G, et al. Genetic control of the CD4/CD8 T-cell ratio in humans. Nat Med 1995;1(12):1279–83.

25. Du Y, Yu K, Yan C, et al. The contributions of Mu-opioid receptors on glutamatergic and GABAergic neurons to analgesia induced by various stress intensities. eNeuro 2022;9(3):ENEURO.0487-21.2022.

26. Osborne NR, Davis KD. Sex and gender differences in pain. Int Rev Neurobiol 2022;164:277–307.

27. Unruh AM. Gender variations in clinical pain experience. Pain 1996;65(2–3): 123–67.

28. Uvelli A, Duranti C, Salvo G, et al. The risk factors of chronic pain in victims of violence: a scoping review. Healthcare (Basel) 2023;11(17):2421.

29. LeResche L. Epidemiology of temporomandibular disorders: implications for the investigation of etiologic factors. Crit Rev Oral Biol Med 1997;8(3):291–305.

30. Bueno CH, Pereira DD, Pattussi MP, et al. Gender differences in temporomandibular disorders in adult populational studies: a systematic review and meta-analysis. J Oral Rehabil 2018;45(9):720–9.

31. Smith SB, Mir E, Bair E, et al. Genetic variants associated with development of TMD and its intermediate phenotypes: the genetic architecture of TMD in the OPPERA prospective cohort study. J Pain 2013;14(12 Suppl):T91-101.e1-3.

32. Ribeiro-Dasilva MC, Peres Line SR, Leme Godoy dos Santos MC, et al. Estrogen receptor-alpha polymorphisms and predisposition to TMJ disorder. J Pain 2009; 10(5):527–33.

33. Xue XT, Zhang T, Cui SJ, et al. Sexual dimorphism of estrogen-sensitized synoviocytes contributes to gender difference in temporomandibular joint osteoarthritis. Oral Dis 2018;24(8):1503–13.

34. Warren MP, Fried JL. Temporomandibular disorders and hormones in women. Cells Tissues Organs 2001;169(3):187–92.

35. LeResche L, Saunders K, Von Korff MR, et al. Use of exogenous hormones and risk of temporomandibular disorder pain. Pain 1997;69(1–2):153–60.

36. Briscoe ME. Why do people go to the doctor? Sex differences in the correlates of GP consultation. Soc Sci Med 1987;25(5):507–13.

37. Robinson ME, Riley JL 3rd, Myers CD, et al. Gender role expectations of pain: relationship to sex differences in pain. J Pain 2001;2(5):251–7.

38. Wise EA, Price DD, Myers CD, et al. Gender role expectations of pain: relationship to experimental pain perception. Pain 2002;96(3):335–42.

39. Tukiainen T, Villani AC, Yen A, et al. Landscape of X chromosome inactivation across human tissues. Nature 2017;550(7675):244–8.

40. Chatzis LG, Goules AV, Tzioufas AG. Searching for the "X factor" in Sjogren's syndrome female predilection. Clin Exp Rheumatol 2021;39 Suppl 133(6):206–14.

41. Rhie A, Nurk S, Cechova M, et al. The complete sequence of a human Y chromosome. Nature 2023;621(7978):344–54.

42. Ross MT, Grafham DV, Coffey AJ, et al. The DNA sequence of the human X chromosome. Nature 2005;434(7031):325–37.

43. Fish EN. The X-files in immunity: sex-based differences predispose immune responses. Nat Rev Immunol 2008;8(9):737–44.

44. Sankaran-Walters S, Macal M, Grishina I, et al. Sex differences matter in the gut: effect on mucosal immune activation and inflammation. Biol Sex Differ 2013; 4(1):10.

45. Sthoeger ZM, Chiorazzi N, Lahita RG. Regulation of the immune response by sex hormones. I. In vitro effects of estradiol and testosterone on pokeweed mitogen-induced human B cell differentiation. J Immunol 1988;141(1):91–8.
46. Kissick HT, Sanda MG, Dunn LK, et al. Androgens alter T-cell immunity by inhibiting T-helper 1 differentiation. Proc Natl Acad Sci U S A 2014;111(27):9887–92.
47. Sarafrazi NS, Wambogo EA, Shepherd JA. Osteoporosis or low bone mass in older adults: United States, 2017-2018. Center for Disease Control, National Center for Health Statistics. NCHS Data Brief 2021;405:1–8.
48. Boyce BF, Xing L. Functions of RANKL/RANK/OPG in bone modeling and remodeling. Arch Biochem Biophys 2008;473(2):139–46.
49. Finkelstein JS, Klibanski A, Neer RM, et al. Osteoporosis in men with idiopathic hypogonadotropic hypogonadism. Ann Intern Med 1987;106(3):354–61.
50. Zhang H, Ma K, Li RM, et al. Association between testosterone levels and bone mineral density in females aged 40-60 years from NHANES 2011-2016. Sci Rep 2022;12(1):16426.
51. National Institutes of Health. Notice Number: NOT-OD-15-102. 2016. Available at: https://grants.nih.gov/grants/guide/notice-files/not-od-15-102.html#:~:text=This%20notice%20focuses%20on%20NIH's,vertebrate%20animal%20and%20human%20studies. Accessed September 10, 2024.
52. Sangalli L, Souza LC, Letra A, et al. Sex as a biological variable in oral diseases: evidence and future prospects. J Dent Res 2023;102(13):1395–416.
53. Martinez-Mier EA, Zandona AF. The impact of gender on caries prevalence and risk assessment. Dent Clin North Am 2013;57(2):301–15.
54. Su S, Lipsky MS, Licari FW, et al. Comparing oral health behaviours of men and women in the United States. J Dent 2022;122:104157.
55. Lipsky MS, Su S, Crespo CJ, et al. Men and oral health: a review of sex and gender differences. Am J Men's Health 2021;15(3):15579883211016361.
56. Clocchiatti A, Cora E, Zhang Y, et al. Sexual dimorphism in cancer. Nat Rev Cancer 2016;16(5):330–9.
57. Smith PH, Bessette AJ, Weinberger AH, et al. Sex/gender differences in smoking cessation: a review. Prev Med 2016;92:135–40.
58. Smith PH, Weinberger AH, Zhang J, et al. Sex differences in smoking cessation pharmacotherapy comparative efficacy: a network meta-analysis. Nicotine Tob Res 2017;19(3):273–81.
59. Verplaetse TL, Morris ED, McKee SA, et al. Sex differences in the nicotinic acetylcholine and dopamine receptor systems underlying tobacco smoking addiction. Curr Opin Behav Sci 2018;23:196–202.
60. American Dental Association. Dental Treatment During Pregnancy (Trans. 2014:508). Current Policies. Last Updated 2023. Page 188. Available at: chrome-extension://efaidnbmnnnibpcajpcglclefindmkaj/https://www.ada.org/-/media/project/ada-organization/ada/ada-org/files/about/governance/current_policies.pdf. Accessed September 10, 2024.
61. Morelli EL, Broadbent JM, Leichter JW, et al. Pregnancy, parity and periodontal disease. Aust Dent J 2018;63:270–8.
62. Hyder T, Khan S, Moosa ZH. Dental care of the pregnant patient: an update of guidelines and recommendations. J Pak Med Assoc 2023;73(10):2041–6.
63. Xiong X, Buekens P, Fraser WD, et al. Periodontal disease and adverse pregnancy outcomes: a systematic review. BJOG 2006;113(2):135–43.
64. American College of Obstetricians and Gynecologists Committee on Health Care for Underserved Women. Oral Health Care During Pregnancy and Through the Lifespan. Reaffirmed 2022. Available at: https://www.acog.org/clinical/clinical-guidance/

committee-opinion/articles/2013/08/oral-health-care-during-pregnancy-and-through-the-lifespan. Accessed September 10, 2024.
65. Black E, Khor KE, Kennedy D, et al. Medication use and pain management in pregnancy: a critical review. Pain Pract 2019;19(8):875–99.
66. Soldin OP, Mattison DR. Sex differences in pharmacokinetics and pharmacodynamics. Clin Pharmacokinet 2009;48(3):143–57.
67. Heinrich J. Drug Safety: Most Drugs withdrawn in recent years had greater health risks in women (GAO-01-286R). Washington, DC: United States General Accounting Office; 2001. Available at: https://www.gao.gov/assets/gao-01-286r.pdf.
68. Niesters M, Dahan A, Kest B, et al. Do sex differences exist in opioid analgesia? A systematic review and meta-analysis of human experimental and clinical studies. Pain 2010;151(1):61–8.
69. Weisse CS, Sorum PC, Sanders KN, et al. Do gender and race affect decisions about pain management? J Gen Intern Med 2001;16(4):211–7.
70. Roter DL, Hall JA, Aoki Y. Physician gender effects in medical communication: a meta-analytic review. JAMA 2002;288(6):756–64.
71. Sandhu H, Adams A, Singleton L, et al. The impact of gender dyads on doctor-patient communication: a systematic review. Patient Educ Counsel 2009;76(3):348–55.
72. Schwartz SB, Sanders AE, Lee JY, et al. Sexual orientation-related oral health disparities in the United States. J Publ Health Dent 2019;79(1):18–24.
73. Fredriksen-Goldsen KI, Kim HJ, Barkan SE, et al. Health disparities among lesbian, gay, and bisexual older adults: results from a population-based study. Am J Public Health 2013;103(10):1802–9.
74. Tharp G, Wohlford M, Shukla A. Reviewing challenges in access to oral health services among the LGBTQ+ community in Indiana and Michigan: a cross-sectional, exploratory study. PLoS One 2022;17(2):e0264271.
75. Macdonald DW, Grossoehme DH, Mazzola A, et al. "I just want to be treated like a normal person": oral health care experiences of transgender adolescents and young adults. J Am Dent Assoc 2019;150(9):748–54.
76. Haley CM and Doubleday AF. Inclusive language to support health equity and belonging in dentistry, Dent Clin N Am, 2024, https://doi.org/10.1016/j.cden.2024.08.001, In Press.
77. Neville BW, Damm DD, Allen CM, et al. Oral and maxillofacial pathology. 5th edition. St. Louis, MO: Elsevier; 2023.

Inclusivity in Mentorship
Shifting Paradigms of Inclusion in Dental Education

Benita N. Chatmon, PhD, MSN, RN, CNE[a],*,
Kendall M. Campbell, MD[b], Charles P. Mouton, MD, MS, MBA[c],
Janet H. Southerland, DDS, MPH, PhD[d],
Leslie R. Halpern, DDS, MD, PhD, MPH, FICD[e]

KEYWORDS

- Mentorship • Inclusive mentorship • Mentorship models • Mosaic mentorship
- Mentorship in dental education • Dentistry

KEY POINTS

- Mentoring involves a developmental relationship where an experienced individual (mentor) guides a less experienced one (mentee) toward mutually defined goals, skill enhancement, career advancement, social and occupational integration, and moral support.
- Different mentoring models include traditional one-on-one (dyadic), peer mentoring, reverse mentoring, group mentoring, e-mentoring, and functional mentoring which encompasses the emerging "mosaic mentoring" model that creates a network of mentors from diverse backgrounds to support various aspects of the mentee's development.
- Inclusive mentoring acknowledges and values the cultural orientation of mentees, addressing biases, stereotype threats, and the need for cultural competence.
- Robust mentoring programs improve recruitment, retention, job satisfaction, and organizational stability in health care and academic settings.
- Addressing cross-cultural communication and mentoring diverse groups is essential for fostering an inclusive and supportive professional environment.

[a] School of Nursing, LSU Health Sciences Center New Orleans, 1900 Gravier Street, New Orleans, LA 70112, USA; [b] Department of Family Medicine, University of Texas Medical Branch, 301 University Drive, Galveston, TX 77550, USA; [c] Family Medicine, School of Medicine, University of Texas Medical Branch, 301 University Drive, Galveston, TX 77550, USA, [d] Oral and Maxillofacial Surgery, Interim Dean of School of Dentistry, LSU Health Sciences Center New Orleans, 433 Bolivar Street, Suite 825, New Orleans, LA 70112, USA; [e] Oral and Maxillofacial Surgery, New York Medical College/ NYC Health + Hospitals/Metropolitan, 1901 First Avenue, New York City, NY 10029, USA
* Corresponding author. 1900 Gravier Street, Off 5B14, New Orleans, LA 70112.
E-mail address: bnwoko@lsuhsc.edu

Dent Clin N Am 69 (2025) 131–144
https://doi.org/10.1016/j.cden.2024.08.009
0011-8532/25/Published by Elsevier Inc.
dental.theclinics.com

INTRODUCTION

Mentoring, a concept deeply embedded in Greek mythology, originated from the story of Odysseus who entrusted his son Telemachus to Mentor, his trusted friend, before leading the army in the Trojan War. Telemachus was guided and advised by Mentor who counseled him during his father's absence.[1] This myth underscores the significance and purpose of mentoring, illustrating its foundational role in guidance and support. The adage "it takes a village" reflects our inherent social nature and desire to help others, a trait particularly strong in health professions. It is within this social framing that mentoring has developed and is the lens through which we can understand how to facilitate its effective application in the academic setting particularly in dentistry.

MENTORING DEFINED AND ITS BENEFIT

In his presidential address to the New York Academy of Medicine in 1995, Jermiah Barondess explored the extensive history of mentoring, highlighting numerous instances across various fields where mentoring relationships have existed.[2] He referenced an early study by Daniel J. Levinson at Yale in 1978, which detailed the multifaceted role of mentors. According to Levinson, mentors are typically older and more experienced, act as teachers, sponsors, advisors, and role models, enhancing mentees' skills, facilitating their career advancement, guiding their social and occupational integration, and providing moral support.[3] Over time, the understanding of these mentoring roles has expanded to include fostering inclusivity and acknowledging diverse perspectives. Modern mentoring now also emphasizes recognizing biases, fostering a sense of belonging, and maintaining respect, all of which contribute to more effective and enriching mentor/mentee relationships.

Mentoring is a 2 way developmental relationship where a more experienced individual guides a less experienced one toward mutually defined goals. It involves sharing knowledge, social capital, and psychosocial support. In academia, mentoring benefits the mentee, mentor, and organization. For mentees, it offers insights, skills, and networks that enhance career growth. Mentors gain satisfaction and professional rejuvenation from guiding the next generation.[4] Organizations benefit through improved recruitment, retention, and a cohesive workforce, essential for high-quality patient care.[5,6]

Benefits for Mentees

Mentees benefit from valuable knowledge specific to their personal and profession goals. Through mentoring, they receive guidance on navigating complex professional landscapes, developing crucial skills, and achieving personal and professional goals. This support system is particularly vital in academic health professions, where the challenges can be multifaceted and demanding.[4,6,7]

Benefits for Mentors

Mentors experience the gratification of guiding the next generation, which can reinforce their own knowledge and skills. This process fosters a sense of fulfillment and professional rejuvenation. Mentors often find that mentoring helps them stay current in their field, enhances their leadership skills, and provides opportunities for personal growth and satisfaction.[4] **Box 1** provides the components that should be considered by the mentor in creating good mentoring experiences.[8]

Benefits for Organizations

Health care organizations reap significant benefits from robust mentoring programs. Effective mentoring enhances recruitment and retention, ensuring a stable and

> **Box 1**
> **Characteristics of good mentoring[8]**
>
> - *Reciprocity:* Ensure equal engagement from both the mentor and the mentee, fostering a balanced and interactive relationship.
> - *Learning:* Focus on acquiring knowledge through active participation and engagement in the learning process.
> - *Relationship:* Establish and maintain trust as the foundation of the mentoring relationship, ensuring both parties feel secure and valued.
> - *Partnership:* Adopt a current paradigm that encourages active involvement and contribution from both partners in the mentoring relationship, promoting mutual growth.
> - *Collaboration:* Engage in the sharing of knowledge, learning together, and building consensus to enhance the mentoring experience.
> - *Mutually defined goals:* Clearly articulate and agree on learning goals to ensure a satisfactory and purposeful mentoring outcome.
> - *Development:* Focus on developing skills, knowledge, abilities, and thinking, guiding the mentee from their current state to their desired future state.

sustainable workforce.[5] This stability not only reduces turnover costs but also cultivates a cohesive and experienced team, which is essential for high-quality patient care. Additionally, a well-supported workforce can lead to improved job satisfaction, reducing burnout, and fostering a positive work environment.[6]

The sustainability of the workforce contributes to a positive organizational reputation, making the institution more attractive to prospective employees and stakeholders. This reputation is crucial in a competitive health care landscape, as it underscores the organization's commitment to professional development and employee well-being.[5] Consequently, mentoring is not just a personal benefit but a strategic organizational asset that promotes long-term success and excellence in academic health professions.

Both health care and academic institutions can greatly benefit from mentoring programs if they intentionally consider the characteristics of effective mentoring programs (**Fig. 1**).[9] Effective mentoring is not a one-size-fits-all approach. It requires careful planning and consideration of several key factors to maximize its benefits.

In this article, various mentoring models, including the emerging mosaic model, are discussed, along with expounding on the inclusive and social construct mentorship framework, addressing the current barriers to mentoring underrepresented groups in the health professions as well as examining the dynamics of the mentoring relationship within the context of dental education. By reinforcing inclusion in dentistry its value will enhance the dental provider workforce across educational research and clinical areas in order to provide a multifaceted approach to foster change.

MENTORING MODELS

Models of mentorship (**Box 2**) can vary based on perceived needs of the mentee, availability, capacity and skillset of the mentor, and the type of mentoring needed. In addition, approaches to the mentoring relationship for someone who may need the inclusion of coaching or sponsorship will be different than someone who may need functional mentoring for a specific project or task.[10–12] According to Halpern, coaching plays a pivotal role in developing the skills and abilities of the mentee. Coaching

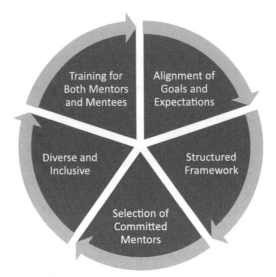

Fig. 1. Characteristics of effective mentoring programs.

focuses on enhancing the mentees' performance aligned with their own specific goals. Coaches are typically well informed, possess strong interpersonal skills, excel in active listening, and foster a judgment-free environment.[13] On the other hand, sponsorship involves advocating for the mentee and increasing their visibility. Unlike mentoring alone, sponsorship carries a higher level of risk.[1] The sponsoring mentor has reputational risks associated with advocating for the mentee should the mentee be unsuccessful. The aim of sponsorship is to extend the advantages of mentorship (such

---

Box 2
Mentoring models[4,14–18]

Mosaic mentoring: Integrates multiple mentoring relationships to address the diverse needs of mentees. This approach leverages different mentors' unique strengths to provide comprehensive support, fostering personal, professional, and academic growth.

Dyadic-traditional one-to-one: A traditional mentoring relationship where one mentor supports one mentee. This model focuses on building a strong, personal connection, allowing for tailored guidance and support based on the mentee's specific needs and goals.

Group/team-based mentoring: Involves multiple mentors and mentees interacting together. This collaborative approach encourages peer learning and support, enhances networking opportunities, and fosters a sense of community and shared learning among participants.

Functional/skill-based mentoring: Focuses on developing specific skills or competencies. Mentors with expertise in particular areas provide targeted guidance and training to help mentees enhance their abilities and achieve their career or academic objectives.

Peer mentoring: Involves individuals at similar stages in their careers or education supporting each other. This model fosters mutual learning and understanding, offering relatable advice and experiences that can be particularly valuable for navigating shared challenges.

E-mentoring: Utilizes digital communication tools to connect mentors and mentees. This model provides flexibility and accessibility, allowing for remote mentoring relationships that can transcend geographic boundaries and offer continuous support through virtual interactions.

as guidance) into the realms where decisions are made (through advocacy) to endorse and support the mentee openly.[14]

Informal mentoring relationships develop organically or through self-selection by either the mentee or mentor. These relationships are characterized by their lack of formal structure or training, with no predetermined goals or outcomes, allowing for flexibility and adaptability as the relationship evolves. Informal mentoring often relies on mutual interests and natural rapport, fostering a more relaxed and fluid dynamic between the mentor and the mentee.[4]

In contrast, *formal mentoring* relationships are highly structured and include specific training and predetermined goals. These relationships are governed by established guidelines or expectations and require a commitment from both the mentor and the mentee. Formal mentoring typically involves a clear framework, including regular meetings, goal-setting sessions, and progress reviews, ensuring that both parties remain focused on achieving the outlined objectives. Both informal and formal mentoring approaches can be effectively integrated into various mentoring models, each offering unique advantages.[4,15]

Traditional one-on-one mentoring, also known as *dyadic or vertical*, where an experienced professional guides a less experienced mentee, provides personalized support and fosters deep, long-term professional relationships. This model was most commonly applied during surgical training in the twentieth century.[16,17] *Peer mentoring*, which pairs students or young professionals at similar stages of their careers, promotes mutual support, and collaborative learning. A senior level faculty mentor may be included. In contrast, *reverse mentoring* connects younger mentors with older mentees to share their knowledge. Most often the knowledge gaps are related to cultural differences and technology innovations.[15]

Group (multiple/constellation/team based) mentoring can involve a single mentor working with multiple mentees or one mentee working with several mentors (the latter is seen most often in Medicine). Group mentoring encourages diverse perspectives and collective problem-solving.[9] *E-mentoring* leverages digital platforms to connect mentors and mentees across geographic boundaries, making mentorship more accessible and flexible. The *functional mentoring* model is project-focused where the mentee is paired with the mentor for a specific skill development or the completion of a project such as the design of a program, grant proposal, or research project.[4,18] These models can be tailored to enhance skills, knowledge, and professional identity considering specific context, goals (research or clinical), and profession. However, the unique challenges in health care necessitate a more inclusive approach.

EVOLUTION TO A "MOSAIC MENTOR"

Based on the above-mentioned models, the *mosaic mentoring* model arose (**Fig. 2**). This approach creates a network of mentors from diverse backgrounds and areas of expertise to support various aspects of the mentee's development. Mosaic mentoring is viewed "as a multi-dimensional guidance and a longitudinal landscape of career mentoring" that includes "a diverse group of individuals of different ranks, ages, genders, races, skills, and experience com[ing] together in a non-hierarchical community or network".[19] Mosaic mentoring can assist the creation of mentoring experiences that acknowledge differences and bridge gaps that may contribute to barriers for individuals underrepresented in medicine from gaining the support that they need to reach their professional goals.

Mosaic mentoring adopts a culturally responsive approach that acknowledges a mentee's cultural orientation to assist in supporting the need and goals of the mentee.

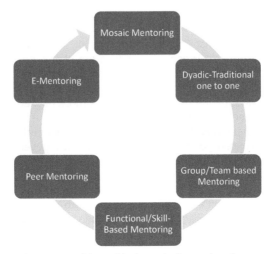

Fig. 2. Mosaic mentoring—a non-hierarchical mentoring network.

Han and colleagues[19] developed and created a mosaic mentoring program for university employees of color and American Indians that involved a culturally responsive mentoring framework. The mission of the program was to adopt a community of support and interconnection to assist members in navigating the university systems, so that members can flourish and reach their goals.

Box 3 describes a model of mosaic mentoring. Read through the vignette to see how mosaic mentoring can be applied into practice.

MENTORING AND THE SOCIAL CONSTRUCT FRAMEWORK

A framework has emerged in the literature where mentoring is viewed through the lens of social capital. Robert Putnam's 1995 publication, "Bowling Alone," describes the collapse of the American community and the need for community in developing mentoring relationships.[20,21] This model of social capital, based on Putnam's essays[21] along with Hanifan's observations in 1916,[22] emphasizes the importance of community in mentoring.

Mentoring requires a level of social interaction involving interpersonal exchanges influenced by both mentee and mentor perceptions.[23] Given the diverse individual attributes and the specific social context (eg, a specific institution, a specific discipline) in which mentoring occurs, successful interaction can lead to culturally informed mentoring relationships.[24] Social capital pertains to the connections among individuals who reside and work within a community, facilitating the effective operation of that community.[25] Let it be proposed that the mentoring process would benefit from application of aspects of the social capital model. This idea was introduced by Hanifan and further expanded by others such as Bourdieu, Carpriano, and Cattell.[26–28] In the context of mentoring, social capital models focus on how relationships and networks contribute to the success and development of individuals and groups. **Table 1** highlights social capital levels and forms, along with some benefits and challenges.

THE EMERGING MODEL OF INCLUSIVITY IN MENTORSHIP

According to Thompson and Taylor, inclusive mentoring involves mentoring across differences by ensuring equitable access to benefits and addressing stereotype

---

Box 3
Vignette for a mosaic mentor model in dentistry

Barbara is a second year dental student who received a scholarship to develop a model for dental rehabilitation in a community of newly arrived immigrants from across the globe. Her interest in global public health made her an ideal candidate for this project. Speaking no other language than English, she knew that community engagement with individuals from these communities was one of the foundational steps for success. She also knew the steps for oral health and wellbeing required an interdisciplinary team approach within and across dental specialties. Her exposure to pre-clinical training in operative, periodontal, endodontics, oral surgery, etc. could be a wonderful set of tools to help her patients.

She listed all of the above and presented her plan to her academic dean who then gathered faculty that would guide her mentorship according to her stated needs. The following were needed:

1. A mentor who could help Barbara navigate the process of communicating with her non-English-speaking patients
2. A mentor who with experience in public health to help her to understand the epidemiology of oral disease in the population she would care for.
3. Several mentors who would guide her in treatment planning based upon the patient needs and desires.
4. Since Barbara was a first-generation leader (in her family) in a health career, she required a mentor that would be of either a gender and/or cultural "mirror" to effectively communicate and collaborate with her patients while understanding/managing her biases and concerns of acceptance by her patient pool. She also needs a mentor for clinical expertise to provide guidance in her role as a dental provider.
5. Barbara's outcomes for success are
   a. Ability to communicate successfully so that her patients trust the role she is playing in their health not only dentally but their overall health.
   b. An improvement in the health and well-being of the community she is serving
   c. Barbara would hope to expand her experiences to other providers so that community engagement will increase the oral health and well-being of future members of the communities they serve.
   d. Another significant outcome would be development of interprofessional health care clinic that provides a patient-centered approach to primary and specialty care in one location.

---

threat, biases, and microaggressions within the mentoring dyad.[1] The inclusive mentorship approach values and appreciates the culture and background of both mentors and mentees. This approach is especially important for underrepresented groups or those with minoritized identities, given the shortage of diversity in the health care workforce. A diverse workforce has been linked to improved patient outcomes and quality performance, amplifying the need for inclusive mentorship experiences.[29] Creating a more inclusive mentoring environment in the specialty of dentistry requires attention to the domains of an inclusive mentoring experience that impact the life of the mentee (**Fig. 3**), one component focusing on the ability to create safety and equity within the mentoring relationship. The domains that may impact the life of a mentee include personal, institutional, and professional life, life as connected to specialty specific societies like the National Dental Association, and life in the context of political, environmental and socioeconomic climates. Appreciating that these domains exist assist in recognizing bias, stereotype threat, and a lack of cultural competence that could exist in a mentoring relationship.

Barriers to inclusive mentorship often stem from traditional approaches that do not adequately recognize or validate the experiences and aspirations of underrepresented groups.[1] Such barriers can include

Table 1
Social capital: levels, forms, benefits and challenges

Levels of Social Capital	Type	Interactions	Benefits
Micro	Networks of individual or groups	Positive or negative	Key role in human capital accumulation, harmony in relationships, stress and risk management
Meso	Involves groups and facilitates collective action	Includes vertical and horizontal associations in behavior	Leverage resources, ideas, and information beyond the community
Macro	Formalized institutional relationships and structures	Political or governmental or social infrastructure	Social wealth, crisis management, relationship between countries

Forms of Social Capital	
Structural	Information sharing and collective action and decision-making through established roles and social networks supplemented by rules, procedures and precedents. (Institutional)
Cognitive	Shared norms, values, trust, attitudes, and beliefs, and is a more subjective and intangible concept. (Relational)

Benefits and Challenges of Social Capital	
Benefits	Challenges
• The norms of reciprocity • Shared values • Interpersonal relationships • Social trust • A shared understanding and identity • Cooperation and collaboration.	• May not be available to all • Can cause social isolation • Can result in exclusion of outsiders • Dependent on socioeconomic position • Can restrict individual freedom.

Data from Bisung E and Elliott SJ. Toward a social capital-based framework for understanding the water health nexus. 2014,108:pp.194-200; and Portes, A. (1998). Social capital: Its origins and applications in modern sociology. Annual Review of Sociology, 24:pp.1-24. https://doi.org/10.1146/annurev.soc.24.1.1.

- *Low mentor expectations*: Mentees from underrepresented groups may face low expectations from their mentors, which can hinder their confidence and progress.
- *Goal misalignment*: A lack of alignment between the goals of the mentor and mentee can lead to frustration and a lack of meaningful progress.
- *Limited motivations for mentorship*: Mentors may not fully understand or appreciate the importance of inclusive mentorship, leading to a lack of genuine investment in the mentee's success.[1]

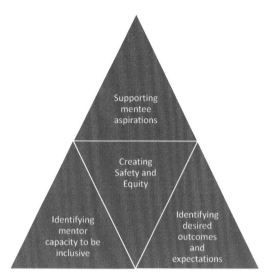

Fig. 3. Domains of inclusive mentoring.

Impacts of mentorship that are not approached from a place of inclusion can be seen as part of the minority tax and a gate blocker to the success and leadership development of the underrepresented minority mentee.[30,31] Adding to the complexities of isolation, diversity efforts and institutional inequities experienced by this group not only impacts the mentee's success, but also disadvantages the institution as it decreases its effectiveness due to decreased investment in employee diversity and strength.[31]

Some strategies for creating inclusive mentoring experiences include defining outcomes and aligning expectations, supporting mentee aspirations, and training for mentors to develop their skills in cross-cultural communication (**Box 4**). When considering mentee's outcomes, the mentor and mentee should agree in the beginning of their relationship on the expectations of the mentoring relationship. Supporting mentee aspirations is also very important.[32,33] Literature shows that faculty who are underrepresented in medicine (UIM) have higher leadership aspirations than their well-represented counterparts.[34,35] These leadership aspirations transfer to any underrepresented minority academician working to support the growth and development of learners while desiring career success and advancement. It is important that mentors recognize and support these aspirations as part of creating an inclusive mentoring experience.

A hidden assumption exists that experience in a profession equates to experience in mentoring. That assumption is false. Training is vital for relationships. Mentors may not understand the complexities of culture or background, but as a mentor they bear the responsibility of learning about and appreciating those things that are of importance to the mentee. Resources are available to assist mentors, including literature on how to work with individuals from different backgrounds to training. Whether unconscious (implicit) or conscious, recognizing the negative impact of bias on the mentorship relationship is a must. Implicit bias can disengage mentees from the mentoring experience, hinder progress, and goal attainment, impact progress in diversifying the scientific workforce and negatively impact health disparities.[36,37] Understanding the diverse backgrounds and perspectives of mentees can bring satisfaction to the

---

Box 4
Strategies for inclusive mentoring[26,27]

- *Defining outcomes and aligning expectations*: The mentor and mentee should agree on outcomes at the start, whether it be to complete a project, compose a manuscript, or create a blueprint for promotion.

- *Supporting mentee aspirations*: Literature shows that faculty who are underrepresented in medicine have higher leadership aspirations than their well-represented counterparts. These leadership aspirations transfer to any underrepresented minority academician working to support the growth and development of learners while desiring career success and advancement. It is important that any mentor recognizes and supports these aspirations as part of being an inclusive mentor.

- *Training for mentors—Developing skills for cross-cultural communication*: Mentoring requires a level of social interaction involving interpersonal exchanges influenced by both the mentee and the mentor perceptions. Given the diverse individual attributes and the specific social context in which mentoring occurs, successful interaction can lead to culturally informed mentoring relationships.

---

mentorship relationship and allow the mentee to thrive. Moreover, appreciating the need for the mentee to "mirror" the community they serve supports the premise of social justice, ensuring that mentorship promotes equitable representation and inclusivity. Moving from cultural competence to cultural intelligence allows the mentor to navigate complex or challenging conversations or experiences around culture or background in a way that promotes the relationship and mentee success.[38]

MENTORING ACROSS DIFFERENCES IN DENTAL EDUCATION

Dentistry along with other health professions historically have leveraged the apprenticeship model as a principal way to prepare the next generation of educators and oral health care professionals. Presently, the model has become more comprehensive with leveraging technology (simulation) and experiential learning opportunities to train students while identifying faculty development opportunities to transition and retain faculty in academic careers. Nevertheless, mentoring in dentistry is facing that existing members of the profession as either dental school faculty members or practicing dentists are less diverse that the students entering dental school or the dental workforce.[39,40] Hence, more deliberate efforts for mentoring are needed as an approach for advancing inclusion in the profession and not to rely on the historical mode of learning effective mentoring skills solely on the job. Mentoring skills are not automatic yet they can be taught and improved.[41]

Mentoring presents an approach that can be used to improve recruitment and retention of dental faculty and to help foster an environment that is inclusive and ultimately diverse. Models of mentoring are traditionally steeped in the academic approach that does not just target the individuals' goals but those of the institution they serve. At times there can be a conflict between the two sets of goals that can limit progress and accomplishment.

The role of the academic institution in creating a nurturing and inclusive environment that fosters effective mentoring opportunities and relationships is pivotal to creating pathways to success for dental professionals. The mentoring process is important for preparation and navigating challenges and barriers to attaining career goals in academia. The building blocks or foundational components that are needed to accomplish this task include trust and safety, diverse perspectives, cultural competence and awareness, mutual respect, learning and growth, retention and success, and opportunities for expanded mentoring networks.

Inclusion in the mentoring space is not without complexity or challenge, but creating the conditions for authentic and meaningful mentoring relationships that manage biases and leverage the important elements outlined will contribute to greater productivity and successes especially for those from marginalized backgrounds. Launching a successful mentoring effort requires good understanding of the goals of the relationship and training. Further, effective mentoring is underpinned by a model described as the "mentor life cycle." This model has several components characterized by (1) a matching process, (2) contracting, (2) use of mentor models or diagnostic tools, (3) appraisal, and (4) peer and group supervision.[5]

While many models incorporate all or some of the components of the mentor life cycle, the need for appropriate training for those serving in a mentoring role is paramount. A significant need is for addressing cross-cultural communication and mentoring dyads or groups that often do not match the cultural identity of the mentee. In this context, the mosaic model becomes particularly important. This model emphasizes the value of diverse perspectives and experiences within the mentoring relationship, fostering an environment where both mentors and mentees can learn from each other. Implementing the mosaic model ensures that mentoring is not only inclusive but also adaptable to the unique cultural backgrounds of each mentee, ultimately enhancing the effectiveness and satisfaction of the mentoring experience.

Ultimately, it is very important for dental and other professionals serving in mentoring roles to understand issues associated with social as well as ethnic/cultural identity development to effectively mentor diverse groups of mentees. Many layers are associated with one's identity and are shaped by societal structures, political powers, environmental exposures, personal experiences as well as others. Understanding culture in the context of the individual and incorporating training on tenets of self-identity, community, and individual needs can help in the preparation of more confident and competent mentors.[42]

SUMMARY

Understanding social and ethnic/cultural identity development is crucial for effectively mentoring diverse groups of mentees. Mentors must recognize the many layers of identity shaped by societal structures, political powers, environmental exposures, cultural identity/competency, and personal experiences. Incorporating training on self-identity, community, and individual needs prepares mentors to be more confident and competent leaders. Inclusive mentoring in dental education is essential for fostering a diverse, supportive, and successful professional environment. By addressing barriers, promoting cultural competence, and creating inclusive mentoring environments, institutions can enhance individual and organizational performance, contributing to the growth and success of underrepresented groups in the health care profession.

CLINICS CARE POINTS

- The role of a mentor has undergone a metamorphosis from the traditional model to a more "mosaic mentor" with innovative strategies specific to the mentee's individual challenges.
- An effective mentor exhibits a degree of seniority, reputation, and experience to enhance the mentee's productivity for success on numerous levels with the alignment of values to ensure long-term success in their disciplines.

- Calls to action are happening to provide formal training of mentors who will become adept in advancing gender equity, diversity, and cultural respect with not only their students, residents, and fellows but also with the patient community.
- Inclusivity in mentorship strives to create a "glue" that melds diversity, equity, and a sense of belonging between the provider and the community they serve.

DISCLOSURES

The authors have nothing to disclose.

REFERENCES

1. Thompson K, Taylor E. Inclusive mentorship and sponsorship. Hand Clin 2023; 39(1):43–52.
2. Barondess JA. A brief history of mentoring. Trans Am Clin Climatol Assoc 1995; 106:1–24.
3. Levinson DJ, Darrow CN, Klein EB, et al. The seasons of a man's life. 1st edition. New York, NY: Alfred A. Knopf; 1978.
4. Henry-Noel N, Bishop M, Gwede CK, et al. Mentorship in medicine and other health professions. J Cancer Educ 2019;34(4):629–37.
5. Nathwani S, Rahman N. Growing in dentistry: mentoring the dental professional. Br Dent J 2022;232(4):261–6.
6. Rasic G, Morris-Wiseman LF, Ortega G, et al. Effective mentoring across differences–best practices and effective models to address the needs of under-represented trainees in surgical residency programs. J Surg Educ 2023;80(9): 1242–52.
7. Nemeth A, Chisty A, Spagnoletti CL, et al. Exploring mentoring experiences, per-ceptions, and needs of general internal medicine clinician educators navigating academia: a mixed-methods study. J Gen Intern Med 2021;36(5):1229–36.
8. Zachary LJ. The mentor's guide: facilitating effective learning relationships. 2nd edition. San Francisco, CA: Jossey-Bass Higher and Adult Education Series; 2013.
9. Johnson J, Bradley K, Bugos K, et al. Mentoring models to support transition to practice programs: one size does not fit all. J Contin Educ Nurs 2024;55(4): 161–4.
10. Schenk L, Sentse M, Lenkens M, et al. Instrumental mentoring for young adults: a multi-method study. J Adolesc Res 2021;36(4):398–424.
11. Marcdante K, Simpson D. Choosing when to advise, coach, or mentor. J Grad Med Educ 2018;10(2):227–8.
12. Sharma G, Narula N, Ansari-Ramandi MM, et al. The importance of mentorship and sponsorship. JACC Case Rep 2019;1(2):232–4.
13. Halpern LR. The odyssey of mentoring. Oral Maxillofac Surg Clin North Am 2021; 33(4):435–47.
14. Thompson K, Taylor E. Inclusive mentorship and sponsorship. Hand Clin 2023; 39(1):43–52.
15. Khatchikian AD, Chahal BS, Kielar A. Mosaic mentoring: finding the right mentor for the issue at hand. Abdominal Radiology 2021;46(12):5480–4.
16. The spiritual mentors of Boethius and Dante: the pagan spirit and the medieval love. Available at: https://johnledinghamprofessional.wordpress.com/2019/12/ 06/the-spiritual-mentors-of-boethius-and-dante-the-pagan-spirit-and-the-medie val-beloved/. Accessed July 12, 2024.

17. Greenberg JA, Jolles S, Sullivan S, et al. A structured, extended training program to facilitate adoption of new techniques for practicing surgeons. Surg Endosc 2018;32(1):217–24.
18. Calaguas NP. Mentoring novice nurse educators: goals, principles, models, and key practices. J Prof Nurs 2023;44:8–11.
19. Han I, Onchwari AJ. Development and implementation of a culturally responsive mentoring program for faculty and staff of color. Interdiscip J Partnersh Stud 2018;5(2):3.
20. Heffron JM. Social capital as mentoring. In: Allen TD, Eby LT, editors. The Wiley International Handbook of mentoring. Hoboken, NJ: Wiley; 2020. p. 29–43.
21. Putnam RD. Bowling alone: America's declining social capital. J Democr 1995; 6(1):65–78.
22. Hanifan LJ. The rural school community centre. Ann Am Acad Pol Soc Sci 1916; 67:130–8.
23. Pfund C, Byars-Winston A, Branchaw J, et al. Defining attributes and metrics of effective research mentoring relationships. AIDS Behav 2016;20(S2):238–48.
24. Allen TD, Eby LT, editors. The Blackwell Handbook of mentoring. Oxford, UK: Blackwell Publishing Ltd; 2007.
25. Andriani L, Christoforou A. Social capital: a roadmap of theoretical and empirical contributions and limitations. J Econ Issues 2016;50(1):4–22.
26. Bourdieu P. Outline of a theory of practice. Cambridge, UK: Cambridge University Press; 1977.
27. Carpiano RM. Toward a neighborhood resource-based theory of social capital for health: can Bourdieu and sociology help? Soc Sci Med 2006;62(1):165–75.
28. Cattell V. Poor people, poor places, and poor health: the mediating role of social networks and social capital. Soc Sci Med 2001;52(10):1501–16.
29. Gomez LE, Bernet P. Diversity improves performance and outcomes. J Natl Med Assoc 2019;111(4):383–92.
30. Amaechi O, Foster KE, Tumin D, et al. Addressing the gate blocking of minority faculty. J Natl Med Assoc 2021;113(5):517–21.
31. Rodríguez JE, Campbell KM, Pololi LH. Addressing disparities in academic medicine: what of the minority tax? BMC Med Educ 2015;15(1):6.
32. National Academies of Sciences, Engineering, and Medicine. The science of effective mentorship in STEMM. Washington, DC: The National Academies Press; 2019.
33. Campbell KM, Rodríguez JE. Mentoring Underrepresented Minority in Medicine (URMM) students across racial, ethnic and institutional differences. J Natl Med Assoc 2018;110(5):421–3.
34. Campbell KM. The diversity efforts disparity in academic medicine. Int J Environ Res Public Health 2021;18(9):4529.
35. Pololi LH, Evans AT, Gibbs BK, et al. The experience of minority faculty who are underrepresented in medicine, at 26 representative U.S. Medical Schools. Acad Med 2013;88(9):1308–14.
36. Javier D, Solis LG, Paul MF, et al. Implementation of an unconscious bias course for the National research mentoring network. BMC Med Educ 2022;22(1):391.
37. Blair IV, Steiner JF, Havranek EP. Unconscious (Implicit) bias and health disparities: where do we go from here? Perm J 2011;15(2):71–8.
38. Sternberg RJ, Wong CH, Kreisel AP. Understanding and assessing cultural intelligence: maximum-performance and typical-performance approaches. J Intell 2021;9(3):45.

39. American dental association. Dentist demographics dashboard. Health policy Institute. 2023. Available at: https://www.ada.org/resources/research/health-policy-institute/us-dentist-demographics. Accessed May 29, 2024.

40. Jones N, Marks R, Ramirez R, et al. Census illuminates racial and ethnic composition of the country. Improved race, Ethnicity Measures show U.S. Is Much more Multiracial. United States Census. Available at: https://www.census.gov/library/stories/2021/08/improved-race-ethnicity-measures-reveal-united-states-population-much-more-multiracial.html. Accessed July 12, 2024.

41. Pfund C, Maidl Pribbenow C, Branchaw J, et al. Professional skills. The merits of training mentors. Science 2006;311(5760):473–4.

42. Batiste H, Denby R, Brinson J. Cross-cultural mentoring in higher education: the use of a cultural identity development model. Mentor Tutoring 2022;30(4):409–33.

Moving?

Make sure your subscription moves with you!

To notify us of your new address, find your **Clinics Account Number** (located on your mailing label above your name), and contact customer service at:

Email: journalscustomerservice-usa@elsevier.com

800-654-2452 (subscribers in the U.S. & Canada)
314-447-8871 (subscribers outside of the U.S. & Canada)

Fax number: 314-447-8029

Elsevier Health Sciences Division
Subscription Customer Service
3251 Riverport Lane
Maryland Heights, MO 63043

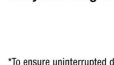

*To ensure uninterrupted delivery of your subscription, please notify us at least 4 weeks in advance of move.

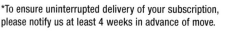

Printed and bound by CPI Group (UK) Ltd, Croydon, CR0 4YY

08/05/2025

01864752-0005